Sensuous Curriculum

Politics and the Senses in Education

A Volume in Landscapes of Education

Series Editors

William H. Schubert
University of Illinois at Chicago
Ming Fang He
Georgia Southern University

Landscapes of Education

William H. Schubert and Ming Fang He, Editors

Sensuous Curriculum: Politics and the Senses in Education (2019)
edited by Walter S. Gershon

Living the Questions: Dispatches From a Life Already in Progress (2017)
by Wade Tillett

From Socrates to Summerhill and Beyond: Towards a Philosophy of Education for Personal Responsibility (2016)
by Ronald Swartz

Necessary Spaces: Exploring the Richness of African American Childhood in the South (2013)
by Saundra Murray Nettles

A Curriculum of Imagination in an Era of Standardization: An Imaginative Dialogue with Maxine Greene and Paulo Freire (2013)
by Robert Lake

Queer South Rising: Voices of a Contested Place (2013)
edited by Reta Ugena Whitlock

Multiliteracies: Beyond Text and the Written Word (2011)
edited by Eugene F. Provenzo, Amanda Goodwin, Miriam Lipsky, and Sheree Sharpe

Listening to and Learning from Students: Possibilities for Teaching, Learning, and Curriculum (2011)
edited by Brian D. Schultz

Love, Justice, and Education: John Dewey and the Utopians (2010)
edited by William H. Schubert

Sensuous Curriculum

Politics and the Senses in Education

edited by

Walter S. Gershon
Kent State University

IAP
INFORMATION AGE PUBLISHING, INC.
Charlotte, NC • www.infoagepub.com

Library of Congress Cataloging-in-Publication Data

CIP record for this book is available from the Library of Congress
http://www.loc.gov

ISBNs: 978-1-64113-581-8 (Paperback)

978-1-64113-582-5 (Hardcover)

978-1-64113-583-2 (ebook)

Printed and bound by CPI Group (UK) Ltd, Croydon, CR0 4YY

CONTENTS

SERIES FOREWORD

LANDSCAPES OF EDUCATION

William H. Schubert and Ming Fang He

In this book series, we explore panoramic landscapes of education. We invite a wide array of authors from diverse theoretical traditions and geographical locations around the world to ponder deeply and critically undulating and evolving contours of educational experience. We perceive contours of educational experience as landscapes that cultivate and are cultivated by who we were and how we become who we are as individuals and as humanity (Nussbaum, 1997). We engage with complex hills and rift valleys, rocky roads and serene pathways, war torn terrains and flowering gardens, towering trees and wuthering grasses, jagged cliffs and unyielding rocks, flowing rivers and uneven oceans evolving with flows of life that shape our perspectives, modify our ideas, and forge our actions. Building upon John Dewey's (1916) *democratic conception of education* and William Schubert's (2009) *ideals of love, justice, and education*, we perceive landscapes of education not only as schools but also as *gathering places* (Dewey, 1933) for humans to pursue worthwhile living. We honor the poetics of landscapes of education flourishing with divergence, convergence, diversity, and complexity of experience.

We look for authors who can move in new directions. We open dialogue on educational issues and situations of shared concerns. We create a space for educational workers such as public intellectuals, scholars, artists, and practitioners to engage in inquiries into education drawn from multiple

Sensuous Curriculum:
Politics and the Senses in Education, pp. vii–xii

perspectives such as art, music, language, literature, philosophy, history, social sciences, and professional studies. We welcome cross-disciplinary, interdisciplinary, transdisciplinary, and counterdisciplinary work. We look for possibilities that are fresh and poetic, nuanced and novelistic, theoretical and practical, personal and political, imaginative and improvisational.

We expand parameters of educational inquiry substantively and methodologically. Substantively, books in this series explore multifarious landscapes wherever education occurs. Such explorations provocatively portray education in schools, workplaces, nonschool settings, and relationships. Methodologically, we encourage diverse forms of inquiry drawing on a wide array of research traditions, approaches, methods, and techniques such as ethnomethodology, phenomenology, hermeneutics, feminism, rhizomatics, deconstructionism, grounded theory, case studies, survey studies, interviews, participant observation, action research, teacher research, activist feminist inquiry, self study, life history, teacher lore, autobiography, biography, memoir, documentary studies, art-based inquiry, ethnography/critical ethnography, autoethnography, participatory inquiry, narrative inquiry, fiction, cross-cultural and multicultural narrative inquiry, psychoanalysis, queer inquiry, and personal~passionate~participatory inquiry (He, Schultz, & Schubert, 2015).

We feature works that amplify the educational value of mass media such as movies, DVDs, television, the Internet, comics, news comedy, cell phones, My Space and Face Book, videos, videogames, computers, and the World Wide Web. We hope to explore how we learn through such electronic frontiers in vastly new ways with little tutelage. We hope to encourage creative improvising, problem posing, critical inquiring, and joyful learning illuminated in these new ways of learning though electronic frontiers which are often suppressed and repressed in schooling. We hope to acknowledge the power of human beings to learn without lesson plans, manuals, worksheets, standardized tests, acquisitive rewards, or external standards.

We encourage expansions that move beyond Western orthodoxies to embrace landscapes from the Eastern (Asian), Southern (African and Latin American), and Oceanic (islandic) worlds. We especially want to see renditions move into *third spaces* (Gutiérrez, Rymes, & Larson, 1995) and *in-between* (He, 2003, 2010) that push boundaries, shift borders, dissolve barriers, and thrive upon contradictions of life. It is our intention that the works featured in this series reveal more of the world-wide landscapes of cultures, ideas, and practices that transgress dominant Western ideologies and their corporate and colonizing legacies. These works have potential in developing transcendent theories of decolonization (e.g., Tuhiwai Smith, 1999/2012), advocating the liberty of indigenous language, cultural rights, and intellectualism (e.g., Grande, 2004), shattering *monocultures of the mind*

(Shiva, 1993), overcoming perils of globalization, and inventing a better human condition for all.

We highlight activist and social justice oriented research (e.g., Ayers, Quinn, & Stovall, 2009) and personal~passionate~participatory inquiry (e.g., He & Phillion, 2008) that engage participation of all citizens, encourage respect, innovation, interaction, cohesion, justice, and peace, and promote cultural, linguistic, intellectual, and ecological diversity and complexity. We celebrate postcolonial feminist work (e.g., Minh-ha, 1989; Mohanty, 2003/2005; Narayan, 1997) that explores migration, slavery, suppression, resistance, representation, difference, race, gender, place, and responses to influential discourses of racism, sexism, classism, and colonialism. We also feature ecofeminist inquiry that explores the intersectionality of repatriarchal historical analysis, spirituality, racism, classism, imperialism, heterosexism, ageism, ableism, anthropocentrism, speciesism, and other forms of oppression (Mies & Shiva, 1993).

Books in this series focus on the what, why, how, when, where, and for whom of relationships, interactions, and transactions that transform human beings to different levels of awareness to build communities and public spaces with shared interests and common goals to strive for equitable, just, and invigorating human conditions. We seek explorations of the educational aspects of relationships (e.g., family, friendship), international, transnational, or intercultural understanding (e.g., exile, diaspora, displacement, indigenous knowledge), and circumstances of living (e.g., poverty, racism, alienation, war, colonization, oppression, and globalization). We want to see how languages, literacies, communities, homes, and families shape images of life's *mysteries and events* (Ulich, 1955), such as love, tradition, birth, death, success or failure, hopes of salvation, or immortality. These educational dimensions of life dynamically influence and are influenced by life in and out of schools (Schubert, 2010) and in-between (He, 2003, 2010). Through engaging such pursuits, this book series illuminates how human beings improvise lives (Bateson, 1989) and commitments in diverse, complicated, and often contested landscapes of education.

Unlike more definitively crafted book series that explicate inclusions and exclusions with ease and precision, our invitations continuously expand. The depths and breadths of landscapes where we live surpass everyday gaze and complicate static analysis. We showcase books that bring a sense of wonder and surprise, make the strange familiar and the familiar strange, and evoke what we do not expect. We do not narrow or define the topics of this series. Rather, we open doors to new perspectives, diverse paradigms, and creative possibilities. We invite authors to surprise us with their insightful ideas of what has been, what is, and what might be.

In this volume, Walter Gershon and a group of creative curriculum scholars continue explorations on sensuous curriculum, politics and senses in education, embarked in the *Journal of Curriculum Theorizing* (Gershon, 2011). The authors featured in this book continue to create a sensuous curriculum (Gershon, 2011, 2018), an innovative form of curriculum inquiry that connects aesthetics and qualitative inquiry with curriculum studies and illuminates the dynamic interactions among bodily praxis, sensual experience of curriculum, and aesthetics of life. Drawing from multiple disciplines such as humanities (e.g., performing arts, philosophy, visual arts), social sciences (e.g., anthropology, cultural studies, geography, political science, sociology), and curriculum studies, Walter Gershon and other authors featured in this book transgress methodological and epistemological boundaries to represent visual, acoustic, and other sensual experience of complicated and contested curriculum that predominantly relies on written languages. These authors have developed innovative lines of inquiry which are grounded in and move beyond such scholarly traditions as sensory and sensual studies (e.g., Howes, 2003, 2005; Stoller, 1997) and curriculum studies (e.g., Au, Brown, & Calderon, 2016; He, Schultz, & Schubert, 2015; Ng-a-Fook, Ibrahim, & Reis, 2016; Paraskeva, 2011; Pinar, Reynolds, Slattery, & Taubman, 1995/2008). These authors call educational workers to transgress boundaries, politicize hopes, liberate potentials, exercise imaginations, and educate senses to fight against all forms of oppression and enact positive educational and social change that fosters equity, equality, freedom, and social justice for all in unjust and contested times.

We applaud with our hearts and souls that the authors featured in this book help us to keep asking central educational questions about what is worthwhile, why, and for whom as we continue to live our lives in an unjust world. They invite us to see that acting upon those questions helps transcend inquiry boundaries, transgress orthodoxy and dogma, dive into the complexities and contradictions of life, embody a particular stance in relation to power, freedom, and human possibility, and promote a more balanced and equitable human condition that embodies cultural, linguistic, and ecological diversities and pluralities of individuals, groups, tribes, and societies conducive to the flourishing of creative capacities that invigorate intellectual, emotional, sensual, moral, and spiritual existence for all.

REFERENCES

Au, W., Brown, A. L., & Calderon, D. (2016). *Reclaiming the multicultural roots of the U.S. curriculum: Communities of color and official knowledge in education*. New York, NY: Teachers College Press.

Ayers, W., Quinn, T., & Stovall, D. (Eds.). (2009). *Handbook of social justice in education*. New York, NY: Routledge.

Bateson, M. C. (1989). *Composing a life*. New York, NY: The Atlantic Monthly Press.

Dewey, J. (1916). *Democracy and education*. New York, NY: Macmillan.

Dewey, J. (1933, April 23). Dewey outlines utopian schools. *New York Times*, p. 7. (Also in Boydston, J. A. (Ed.), *The later works (1925–1953) of John Dewey*, Volume 9, (pp. 136–140) Carbondale, IL: Southern Illinois University Press, 1989.)

Gershon, W. S. (Ed.). (2011). Sensual curriculum: Understanding curriculum of and through the senses. [Special Issue] *Journal of Curriculum Theorizing, 27*(2).

Gershon, W. S. (Ed.). (2018). *Sound curriculum: Sonic studies in educational theory, method, & practice* (Studies in Curriculum Theory Series). New York, NY: Routledge.

Grande, S. (2004). *Red pedagogy: Native American social and political thought*. New York, NY: Rowman & Littlefield.

Gutiérrez, K. D., Rymes, B., & Larson, J. (1995). Script, counterscript, and underlife in the classroom: James Brown versus Brown v. Board of Education. *Harvard Educational Review, 65*(3), 445–471.

He, M. F. (2003). *A river forever flowing: Cross-cultural lives and identities in the multicultural landscape*. Greenwich, CT: Information Age Publishers.

He, M. F. (2010). Exile pedagogy: Teaching in-between. In J. A. Sandlin, B. D. Schultz, & J. Burdick (Eds.), *Handbook of public pedagogy* (pp. 469–482). New York, NY: Routledge.

He, M. F., & Phillion, J. (2008). *Personal~passionate~participatory inquiry into social justice in education*. Charlotte, NC: Information Age Publishing.

He, M. F., Schultz, B. D., & Schubert, W. H. (Eds.). (2015). *The SAGE guide to curriculum in education*. Thousand Oaks, CA: SAGE.

Howes, D. (2003). *Sensual relations: Engaging the senses in culture & social theory*. Ann Arbor, MI: University of Michigan Press.

Howes, D. (Ed.). (2005). *Empire of the senses: The sensual culture reader* (Sensory Formations). New York, NY: Berg.

Mies, M., & Shiva, S. (1993). *Ecofeminism*. Halifax, Nova Scotia, Canada: Fernwood.

Minh-Ha, T. T. (1989). *Woman, native, other: Writing postcoloniality and feminism* (Midland Books). Bloomington, IN: Indiana University Press.

Mohanty, C. T. (2005). *Feminism without borders: Decolonizing theory, practicing solidarity*. Durham, NC: Duke University Press. (Original work published 2003)

Narayan, U. (1997). *Dislocating cultures: Identities, traditions, and third world feminism*. New York, NY: Routledge.

Ng-a-Fook, N., Ibrahim, A., & Reis, G. (2016). *Provoking curriculum studies: Strong poetry and arts of the possible in education*. New York, NY: Routledge.

Nussbaum, M. (1997). *Cultivating humanity: A classical defense of reform in liberal education*. Cambridge, MA: Harvard University Press.

Paraskeva, J. M. (2011). *Conflicts in curriculum theory: Challenging hegemonic epistemologies*. New York, NY: Palgrave Macmillan.

Pinar, W. F., Reynolds, W. M., Slattery, P., & Taubman, P. M. (2008). *Understanding curriculum: An introduction to the study of historical and contemporary curriculum discourses*. New York, NY: Peter Lang. (Original work published 1995)

Schubert, W. H. (2009). *Love, justice, and education: John Dewey and the Utopians*. Charlotte, NC: Information Age Publishing.

Schubert, W. H. (2010). Outside curriculum. In C. Kridel (Ed.), *Encyclopedia of curriculum studies* (pp. 624–628). Thousand Oaks, CA: SAGE.

Shiva, V. (1993). *Monocultures of the mind: Perspectives on biodiversity and biotechnology.* Atlantic Highlands, NJ: Zed Books.

Smith, L. T. (2012). *Decolonizing methodologies: Research and indigenous peoples.* London, England: Zed Books. (Original work published 1999)

Stoller, P. (1997). *Sensuous scholarship* (Contemporary Ethnography). Philadelphia, PA: University of Pennsylvania Press.

Ulich, R. (1955). Response to Ralph Harper's essay. In N. B. Henry. (Ed.), *Modern philosophies of education*, Fifty-fourth Yearbook (Part I) of the National Society for the Study of Education (pp. 254–257). Chicago, IL: University of Chicago Press.

INTRODUCTION

ARTICULATING SENSUOUS CURRICULA

Walter S. Gershon
Kent State University

The sensuous is the human experience. It inscribes the contours of our everyday experiences and articulates our affect. Without sensory information and the normalized values of a sensorium, we could not know, be, or do. For we gain information of our worlds through our senses and interpret that information through our perceptions, the sociocultural patterns individuals and groups utilize to analyze that input. This is the case regardless of how one constructs the sensorium, from a more limited Western five senses model to more complex constructions (e.g., Guerts, 2002; Howes, 2009; Smith, 2012). It is also the case irrespective of divisions between the senses, the locus of their expression, or the ways in which they are understood to function. Further, because there are often greater differences between members within a particular group than divergences between groups, how one attends to and acts on the sensory is always a polyphonic tapestry constructed on the warp of the sociocultural and the weft of individualism. Education, the transfer of information between people, animals, things, and ecologies, is a sensory endeavor.

Sensual curriculum (Gershon, 2011) is one means of enunciating this deeply layered nexus of what I call educational ways of beingknowingdoing

Sensuous Curriculum:
Politics and the Senses in Education, pp. xiii–xx

(Gershon, 2017), the inseparable connections that underscore the notion that being involves knowing, knowing involves being, and both being and knowing are an always already ongoing emergent action of doing something. An understanding of education as sensuous speaks at once to deep histories of educational scholarship (e.g., Cooper, 1892; Dewey, 1998/1934; DuBois, 1903; Truth, 1855; Woodson, 1933) and a (re)emerging attention to the affectively ontological in curriculum studies (e.g., Andreotti, 2011; Gershon, 2013a, 2017; Powell, 2010; Springgay & Freedman, 2012). Its construction at once expresses possibilities voiced in interdisciplinary fields such as affect theory, (new) materialisms, performance studies, critical area studies, post-next methodologies and theories, sensory studies, and sound studies, while attending to questions central to contemporary educational scholarship including those that regard processes of power, positionality, identity, context, and content. Additionally, the notion that the senses and the sensuous as central is somehow "new" not only overlooks many deep educational histories but also in many ways ignores non-Western, Indigenous, non-Christian conceptualizations of the complex intersection between people, ecologies, processes, affect, and embodied knowledges (e.g., Gershon, 2016).

For example, although it is not necessarily framed in this fashion, a central reason that both critical Black intellectual traditions and Indigenous traditions are often marginalized in mainstream U.S. scholarship, and women and queer peoples and groups within those traditions further marginalized, is due to their foregrounding of the affect, ontology, and the senses. Their marginalization is many ways the result of Eurocentric understandings that are often tied to lingering Enlightenment ideas and ideals that nonetheless remain in many constructions of new materialisms and post-qualitative perspectives—understandings that tend to falsely elevate the primacy of knowledge (of and centered in the mind), text, and the ocular (Gershon, 2013, 2017). In no small part, it is a focus on the ocular that makes *framing* ideas both possible and paramount, creates conditions to decouple and devalue feelings and the affectively ontological, and provide a foundation to *see* difference as deficit or interpret a lack of notation as an absence of intelligence (Gershon, 2011, 2017).

Such moves are possible because, while sensory input can be construed as value-neutral—although this too is certainly debatable and a perspective with which I completely disagree—perception, interpretations of that input, is always necessarily value-laden. Similarly, although one's ability to gather sensory information is person-dependent—only you hear the way you hear due to the unique combination of physical structures and processes that are yours and yours alone—the interpretation of that information is never only yours. Where a sharp loud popping sound is informational, its immediate interpretation as a car backfiring, a boat starting, a tree branch falling, or a gun firing is sociocultural and experiential.

Additionally, because people always filter sensory information they receive through multiple layers of sociocultural norms and values in order to make sense, the sensuous is inexorably political. The fields of understanding through which a sensorium is constructed and interpreted always regard questions of *whose* values are in play and what is considered normal to *whom*. Sensuous understandings therefore have material consequences. The ways in which contemporary education functions as a school-to-prison pipeline for young males of color, the exponential difference in suicide rates for queer youth, and continuing gender disparities in science education for girls are but three examples of such consequences.

Further, these understandings are a complicatedly braided knot in which it is entirely possible for (1) a person to be ostracized within a given group for ascribing to broader norms and values or (2) to be marginalized for resonating with local ways of being that clash with only slightly less local ontologies. Or, as but one of many possible everyday examples that a biracial female student at my predominantly white institution once shared with me in frustration: "I'm damned if I do, and screwed if I don't. I'm too light for the Black students, too dark for the white students, and both groups definitely trip when they hear I'm going to be a science teacher."

It is in these and other such ways that people affect and are affected as much by their ecologies as one another, all of which contribute in some fashion to their ever-increasing knowledges. As such, affects are educational, ontologies are the contexts in which our knowleges are born and raised, and the sensuous is as irrevocably embedded in the epistemological as it is in the ontogenic.

Contributions to this edited book deepen and expand upon previous constructions of sensual curriculum, that I now refer to as sensuous curriculum,[1] particularly as outlined in a special issue of the *Journal of Curriculum Theorizing* dedicated to this topic. In it, I located sensual curriculum at the intersection of sensory and curriculum studies, stating that, "this special issue has something to contribute to both fields, the enunciation of the sensual in curriculum studies and a broadening of definitions for curriculum in sensory studies" (Gershon, 2011, p. 1). Not unlike this book, the special issue addressed several of the key points raised above.

However, contributions to that volume tended to talk about ontologies but focus on epistemologies, attend to questions of effects over affects, and implied the necessity of textual explications to render non-textual information sensible. In response to these tendencies and reflecting continuing developments in scholarship of the senses across the multiplicities of its forms and expressions, this book more seeks to more expressly enunciate blossoming possibilities at a node of sensuous methodologies, theories, and their expressions in education.

In short, the purpose of this book is to provide a few concrete points to delineate a field of study called sensuous curriculum in ways that both outline its contours and trace some of its topographies. Neither contributing colleagues nor I in my role as editor seek to create anything resembling standards or rules about these boundaries with one exception. Unlike some forms of arts-based, aesthetic, and other visual and performing arts oriented forms of scholarship, as noted above, sensuous curriculum follows a now-decades old understanding in the social sciences that no strong scholarship can exist without somehow attending to questions of power. To clarify, this is not a Marxist reading, rooted in any particular tradition, or a not-so-subtle attempt to re-anthropomorphize scholarship in the face of a rising tide of new materialisms on one hand and Indigenous understandings on the other (e.g., Ares, Buendia & Helfenbein, 2017; Tuck & MacKenzie, 2015). Instead, it is a recognition that a lack of attention to the processes and structures in which humans are involved—be they understated or overt, focused on persons, objects, or other ecological features, and regardless of their fluidity or the porousness of their boundaries—relates in some fashion to questions about equity, accessibility, liberation, and justice.

Additionally, it is a work in which we acknowledge that language falls short. Sometimes things need to be heard to be understood and are conceptualized in your solar plexus. It is an articulation that queering our perceptions should be the norm for social sciences, in many ways, as it has been for at least the past 40 years. For example, how else are we to understand the Spindler and Spindler (1982) explanation that a central purpose of (educational) anthropology is to make the familiar strange and the strange familiar? This book underscores the kinds of ideals, ideas, and processes that are lost when our scholarship misses sensation for signification or overlooks the ontological in our quest to better articulate the epistemological.

Finally, in our post-next conceptualizations built on blooming (Greigg & Seigworth, 2010, p. 10) and sticky (Ahmed, 2010, p. 230) affects, crunchy ontologies, and flowing epistemologies, we are again pressing at the possibilities for what curriculum might be and how it can function. While not always acknowledged in this fashion, "curriculum" within the field of curriculum studies is often expressed as follows:

- Formal curriculum, the knowledges students are intended to learn in schools (textbooks, assessments)
- Hidden curriculum, the often implicit norms and values expressed through both everyday interactions and in the formal curriculum

- Enacted curriculum, the meanings and understandings educational actors create together through their everyday interactions
- Delivered curriculum, the information teachers present to their students through pedagogy (how teachers teach)
- Null curriculum, noticeable for its absence (the gay rights movement in most high school social studies classes)

Although it is certainly the case that there is some overlap between these curricular forms, contributions to this book suggest further blurring of such lines as well as perhaps new kinds of curriculum, a curriculum of affect for example.

What makes these works so strong, and what makes curriculum so significant, is that it provides a means for the critical examination of educational ecologies and interactions within and outside of formal institutions such as schools. How one passes information between people, the ways in which one learns from objects and environments, how animals teach people about love, and the ways that machines can render the complex sensible are all questions of curriculum. In addition, as noted in the opening paragraph, because the senses are always located in the distinctly individual and the socioculturally contextualized, sensuous curriculum simultaneously speaks to the complexity of curriculum and its imbricated sociocultural contexts. Such understandings also underscore the never-finished, always-emergent nature of beingknowingdoing. Tasting curriculum, inspecting ontologies, smelling knowledges.

Then there are the chapters. They have been organized to accent particular resonances (Gershon 2013b, 2013c, 2017) but can be approached in any order. As I have suggested elsewhere, the strength in such post-structural (or post-post-structural as the case may be) constructions is that they simultaneously create the space for points of convergence between at first disparate-seeming possibilities while allowing divergences to vibrate alone without a need for reconciliation in order to be recognized as valuable. I have elected to document them here in numerical order to more transparently render my own reasoning for their placement rather as than a somehow subversive attempt to encourage such a linear pathway to be followed or any form of correctness in the making. I continue to wrestle with their placement. This is the pleasure of working with such a strong, vibrant group of scholars—each chapter is a complete argument that combines to create a messy, complex, braided whole that folds in and around itself in an endlessly iterative and recursive fashion.

The work opens with critical questions about knowledge, order, and the senses. Bernadette Baker's examination of the roles that the sensorium might play in the politics of knowledge is followed by David Carlson and Joe Sweet who utilize aspects of Michel Foucault and Julia Kristeva's theoretical undertakings to consider relationships between the subject, history, and how one makes sense as well as the possibilities for nonsense.

This leads to Lee Airton's chapter that puts its scholarly finger on the pulse of a longstanding question about language and politics as they wonder about possibilities and limits for an affective "social justice curriculum": Do we need the words to do the work? Approaching similarly incisive questions of affect from another trajectory, Boni Wozolek's chapter focuses on how communities of color can be understood as resistant responses to the affects of racism and racist education for traditionally marginalized youth in school.

Pursuing critical questions at intersections of Blackness and education, Valerie Kinloch and Carlotta Penn articulate how a Black sensuality might be valuable not only in theory and praxis but also as an interruption to whiteness and oppression in schools. Next, Avi Lessing takes on what he calls the visceral curriculum, the complex nexus of bodily experiences of teachers and students through the lens of his own embodied experiences. Echoing themes of the roles of language and identities present in the previous two chapters from yet another pathway, Awad Ibrahim speaks to a sensuous curriculum of investment and its potential as a more equitable and accessible means for examining Black youth and culture.

The final chapters of this edited volume begin with my textually performative critique that moves across vantage points to affectively argue for what I call the ontological problem of contemporary education in the United States. Kim Powell and Sue Uhlig then utilize their experiences with a course in sensory ethnography to argue for arts-based research as a means to consider sensuous questions surrounding a curriculum of place. In the book's concluding chapter, Anniina Souminen moves from questions of research to everyday education to examine the possibilities and potential of attention to pl/sp/aces for both those conceptualizing and engaged in educational interactions.

As is likely evident to the reader, these chapters tack back and forth between theory and practice, slide across scales of method, location, and positionality, and are all deeply invested in notions of social justice. Pressing on the point made above about the strength and order of chapters, contributions to this book combine to document the deep theoretical and practical potential for sensuous curriculum while creating a sum that is truly something more than their excellent composite arguments. Chapters in this edited volume resonate within and across each other not only thematically but also across multitude of layers of the sensorium, affectively articulating the power of the sensuous and its inherent simultaneity. Like a *griot*, they speak of history and now, neither/nor/both/and/beyond, the impossibility of separation and the utterly messy nature of place/people/things/ecologies, and smack a body with potential.

In sum, as these chapters help make plain, there are unending variations to the sensory and their use in theory, method, and practice, within and outside of education. These understandings underscore the necessarily political nature of perceptions, the significance of the sensorium in all aspects of anything that might be called education, and further open the doors for explorations in/as/through/around sensuous curriculum. Sensuous curriculum brings such possibilities to the fore and encourages their exploration in ways that locate it as central to curriculum studies while providing myriad tools for pushing at its boundaries and interrupting the ongoing construction of normalcies in the field. For, in the end, our lives are always sensuous in all their possible iterations and, therefore, so is anything that might be called education.

NOTE

1. This change in working is due to some of the pushback received for the baggage that can accompany the construct of "sensual," within the field of sensory studies, primarily around potentially sexist and misogynist understandings of the sensuous as tied to various forms of sexualization/othering of girls and women. As this work is tied to questions of politics, power, and social justice, I have changed the naming of the work in order to remove the possibility of misinterpretation along these lines, another way in which this volume builds upon the special issue of JCT in 2011.

REFERENCES

Ahmed, S. (2010). *The promise of happiness.* Durham, NC: Duke University Press.

Andreotti, V. (2011). *Actionable postcolonial theory in education.* New York, NY: Palgrave.

Ares, N., Buendia, E., & Helfenbein, R. (Eds.). *Deterritorializing/reterritorializing: Critical geographies of educational reform.* Rotterdam, the Netherlands: Sense.

Cooper, A. J. (1892). *A voice from the south (by a black woman from the south).* Xenia: OH: Aldine Printing House.

Dewey, J. (1998). *Art as experience.* New York, NY: Perigree. (Original work published 1934)

DuBois, W.E.B. (1903). *The souls of Black folk.* Chicago, IL: McClurgand.

Gershon, W. S. (Ed.). (2011). Sensual curriculum: Understanding curriculum of and through the senses. [Special Issue]*Journal of Curriculum Theorizing, 27*(2).

Gershon, W. S. (2013a). Vibrational affect: Sound theory and practice in qualitative research. *Cultural Studies ←→ Critical Methodologies, 13*(4), 257–262.

Gershon, W. S. (2013b). Resonance, affect, and ways of being: Implications of sensual curriculum for educational theory and urban first graders' literacy practices. *The Journal of School and Society.* Retrieved from http://jds.wabash.edu/jds/journal/current-issue/volume-1-issue-1-august-2013/featured-article/

Gershon, W. S. (2013c) Resounding science: A sonic ethnography of an urban fifth grade classroom. *Journal of Sonic Studies*, *4*(1). Retrieved from http://journal.sonicstudies.org/vol04/nr01/a08

Gershon, W. S. (2016). The sound of silence: The material consequences of scholarship. In N. Snaza. S. E. Truman, D. Sonu & Z. Zowiska (Eds.), *Pedagogical matters: New materialisms and curriculum studies*. New York, NY: Peter Lang.

Gershon, W. S. (2017). *Sound curriculum: Sonic studies in educational theory, method, and practice*. New York, NY: Routledge.

Geurts, K. L. (2002). *Culture and the senses: Bodily ways of knowing in an African community*. Berkeley, CA: University of California Press.

Gregg, M., & Seigworth, G. J. (2010). *The affect theory reader*. Durham, NC: Duke University Press.

Howes, D. (Ed.). (2009). *The sixth sense reader*. Oxford, England: Berg Press.

Powell, K. (2010). Making sense of place: Mapping as a multisensory research method. *Qualitative Inquiry*, *16*(7), 539–555. doi:10.1177/1077800410372600

Smith, L. T. (2012). *Decolonizing methodologies: Research and indigenous people* (2nd ed.). London, England: Zed Books.

Spindler, G., & Spindler, L. (1982). Roger Harker and Schönhausen: From the familiar to the strange and back again. In G. Spindler (Ed.), *Doing the ethnography of schooling: Educational anthropology in action* (pp. 20–47). New York, NY: Holt, Rinehart, & Winston.

Springgay, S., & Freedman, D. (2012). *Mothering a bodied curriculum: Emplacement, desire, affect*. Toronto, Canada: University of Toronto Press.

Truth, S. (1851). A'int I a woman? Retrieved from http://www.nps.gov/wori/historyculture/sojourner-truth.htm

Tuck, E., & McKenzie, M. (2015). *Place in research: Theory, methodology, and methods*. New York, NY: Routledge.

Woodson, C. G. (1933). *The mis-education of the Negro*. Retrieved from https://historyisaweapon.com/defcon1/misedne.html

CHAPTER 1

ACTIVATE OR EVACUATE TO EDUCATE?

Roles of a Sensorium in Debates Over Onto-Epistemology

Bernadette M. Baker
University of Wisconsin

INTRODUCTION

> with his hands he [man] writes laws, erects temples and statues, constructs vessels, makes flutes, harps, knives, pincers, and all instruments needed in the arts. It is by them, that he transmits his meditations to posterity, just as, at the present moment, he can converse with Plato, Aristotle, and Hippocrates. The hands, therefore, were most suitable to man, as an intelligent being; for, he is not the most intelligent being because he has two hands as Anaxagoras maintains; but, he is provided with hands because he is the most intelligent; as Aristotle had already, with reason, advanced. It is not the hands, which have taught men the arts; but it is his understanding. (Gall, 1835, p. 124)

Sensuous Curriculum:
Politics and the Senses in Education, pp. 1–28

In discourses identified today as Western educational theory-practice, constructivist, learner centered pedagogy is positioned as a sensitive, tolerant and progressive way to engage children and youth in formal classroom settings. Placing the nature and the needs of the learner at the center of instructional design, supporting students to maintain an active rather than passive orientation to curriculum, and participating in a co-construction that occurs when teachers and learners can readily switch or blend roles is thought to generate something better, higher quality, more desirable, more democratic or more effective. The past implied by learner-centered and constructivist approaches appears in contrast dry rather than fluid, one of sovereign power, direct instruction, static positions, and unbending rules. The image called up further conjoins teacher-centered didactics with a particular version of curriculum—timeless content, universal examination, little consideration of contextual differences, and a potential deadening achieved through repetition of content and form. In such a caricature of direct instruction, authority and knowledge are considered both centralized and transparent, embodied in the pedagogical leader, the child is therefore always the learner, never one who teaches, and the test is considered objective, informative, and efficient, fulfilling its sorting function in meritocratic ways that reflect the ability and effort of the student.

Integral to images of constructivist, learner-centered pedagogy is the blur effected between ontology and epistemology. Onto-epistemology references the suspension of automatic or presumed divisions, drawing attention to the ambiguity and uncertainty between a definitive who and what, between producer and product, between teacher and learner, between subject and environment. The ambiguity is achieved in part through the unspoken leverage given to multisensory and multimodal engagement, formative rather than summative assessment, and the ownership taken over the contextual drivers of performance in the classroom by all of its members, changing what is evaluated or what matters along the way. This is a somewhat different milieu for engagement than that implied by direct instruction models. In direct instruction, the senses are allocated a role primarily of absorbing teachers' directions, enacting obedience to commands, and imitating content. In this frame where student performance is measured largely by final tests the sensorium becomes buried as instrumentally enabling the reception of instruction and the formation of answers.

While such caricatures of pedagogical settings are readily available in teacher education and curriculum studies literature, they are also somewhat disingenuous in regard to the messy enactments integral to many classrooms. The binarization, while instructive for teacher education novices, can minimize the overlap, interpenetration, variety, complexity, and combinatorial potentials of pedagogical acts that often do not draw fully, cleanly, or neatly from any one philosophy or approach. Further, such binarization as teacher centered versus learner centered can obscure that which makes such stylizations two sides of the same coin. For example, even while the number and role of the sensorial pathways involved in traditional teacher centered approaches appears relatively limited, both pedagogical styles directly and indirectly invoke appeal to a sensorium for some kind of claim that makes education, however defined, seem possible and desirable. The senses are naturalized and involved in different ways, required to fulfill certain functions within somewhat different philosophical frames, yet they meet up in the presumption of the material-empirical-sensorial that undergirds the habits of education-as-schooling.

Particularly central to those habits are discourses of vision that draw upon broad, multifarious and longstanding debates in Western philosophy over relationships between vision, seeing, truth, knowledge production, and being.[1] For instance, where assessment and sorting are concerned, despite the disconnect often assumed between constructivist, learner centered pedagogy and direct instruction, teacher centered models, in both cases assessment and sorting could not take place at all without the presumption at a minimum of a sighted observer and the observed. The provincialism of such a seeming obviousness is exposed more fully, however, when one considers that other possibilities have and do exist in archives within and beyond "Western" ones, such as the revelationist onto-epistemologies of Platonic cosmology in Western pasts or the necessary evacuation of the play of the senses in contemporary Buddhist versions—"Eastern" and "Western"—of ultimate Truth (as opposed to conventional, daily, or pragmatic truths).[2] In both examples, the interior/exterior line around the human is less clear, while appeal to an environment and/or outside observer could also be construed as part of a problem or as a weakness. In such cases, appealing to something perceived as exterior or "in the environment" or checking in with an "outside observer" would not operate as sources of authority or verification. To make these moves analytically would operate instead as signs of intellectual dependency, misunderstanding, and/or illusion.

This chapter thus analyzes how roles attributed to a sensorium shape and are shaped by philosophical debates connected to education (and its shifting definition and practice) that generate flashpoints in ontology, epistemology and onto-epistemology. Instead of pitting learner centered against teacher centered or activation against evacuation, however, this chapter analyzes a basic example of the *mobilization* of philosophical provincialism at a pivotal moment in Western thought. It examines in particular how the politics of the senses were tied to the politics of knowledge production through the materialist phrenological reasonings of the 19th century.

Phrenology, the science and art of squeezing the head and analyzing the cranium (thought of as multiple organs of the brain) to describe people's propensities, talents and faults, while now discredited as pseudo-science and fad, has bequeathed systems of reasoning that still haunt the educational field. It is not a coincidence that phrenology took greatest hold as a theory and demonstration in those geopolitical locations that constructed and favored whiteness and masculinity. F. J. Gall (1758–1828) was considered the father of phrenology in the late eighteenth and early 19th centuries in Europe and the United Kingdom, with his writing spreading to the more northern parts of the north American continent and to British and European colonies over the 1800s. His work was popularized and spread with zeal in his own time, as well as mocked, while today it is considered highly offensive for good reason, promoting as it does in subtle and overt ways belief in castes of educability. As the opening quote suggests, it is not that the senses, such as touch and the hands, were not considered useful or enabling. It was that for Gall they were not *determining*—something else sat at the origin, driving the differentiation evident in populations and species, which the hands then simply enacted. I will revisit here, then, Gall's challenge to more widely accepted versions of a sensorium in his own time and how this challenge constituted a specific version of determinism and a particular definition of education.

Gall focused especially on linking perceived differences in "the moral and intellectual faculties" to notions of the inborn, yet the senses still had a role to play. While much of the way in which discourses of race, sex, ability, criminality and more have operated through Gallian texts, what an analysis of their arguments can alert educational fields such as teacher education and curriculum studies to is the artfulness in and availability of how appeal to "the senses" can be taken up as a rationalization for many, even oppositional belief systems. I suggest here that this is not because of the universality of a unique human sensorium or claims to "its" perceived utilitarian, adaptationist or evolutionary necessity, but rather a function of particular Western conceptions of being and knowledge that have come to privilege materiality as a condition of proof and conduit to reason's unfoldment and/or building. This alertness gives pause for thought regarding the naturalization of the senses that heavily psychologized versions of Western teacher education especially seem to rely on, whether promoting learner or teacher centered instruction. It thus points both curriculum studies and teacher education toward a deeper consideration of the potential baggage that particular worldviews can embody, even where well-intended claims to the active, the agentive, the constructivist, and the participatory are launched as automatic moral goods.

POLITICS OF THE SENSES

In what is now described as learner centered pedagogy Rousseau's novella, Émile *ou De l'éducation,* has been positioned as one of the most significant texts in the field of Western educational theory (Wokler, 1995). Generating hostile and positive reactions from his contemporaries, from banning and burning to translation into multiple languages, it accrued its reach in part from the ways in which it was subsequently redeployed in narratives about the emergence of child centeredness (Baker, 2001a). Child centeredness, rather than learner centeredness, implied a certain sensitivity toward the young as unique subjects with their own nature and needs and as beings who could display willful Wills that needed to be managed artfully and tenderly within a social contract. As Émile is tutored in the earlier years of life, for instance, both corporal punishment and reasoning with young children are equally banished (Rousseau, 1977). Neither is considered an appropriate rearing or shaping strategy, yet if the tutor (or today the teacher or parent) cannot hit the child *or* use language appropriate to the child's level of understanding and thereby reason with the child, then what pedagogical strategies are left? How is obedience or understanding procured without hitting on the one hand or verbally explaining why the answer might be "No" on the other? Into this vacuum, modeling and "indirect" forms of pedagogy stepped. Their eventual elevation relied in part on attaching a conception of reason-morality to constructs called knowledge, attaching knowing to a conception of experience, and experience to the operation of a sensorium—broadly posited in Émile as portals through which modeling and instruction would be perceived and objects or things engaged.

To depict Émile as primarily concerned with teaching techniques and pedagogical arts, however, would be to miss the enormity of what framed its controversy and innovation (Baker, 2001b). This included vociferous debate over religion, Rousseau's disdain for organized forms of Christianity, and his preference for "natural religion." In Émile, Rousseau makes appeal to the senses as part of the logic used to undermine reliance upon a Catholic conception of Original sin as the inborn, the internal, or the at-birth-equals-the-innate. While Rousseau does not deny some kind of (changing) human essence in what he saw as Man living in (degraded) civilizations, he does not describe that essence as sin. In such a framing, the activity attributed to a sensorium does not emerge or operate as neutral and its proximity to the term natural or role in enabling "natural religion" does not make a sensorium an innocent or value-free reference point.

In contrast to the furor over Émile and controversy over the role of the senses in Rousseau and in Lockean epistemology before him, in much contemporary educational discourse, especially teacher education research inspired by psychology, the organized activation of the senses and approaches such as learner centered pedagogy, which trade on the multisensory and multimodal, are generally positioned as automatic goods, as ahistorical and contextless, yet as suited to modern educational times. There seems little engagement with existing bodies of research that both historicize the politics of the senses and that question claims to value-neutrality. For example, research now associated with the humanities and religious studies has debated the sensorium as an overtly political site for centuries, contemporary disability studies literature has contested ableist subjectivities that have emerged around sense-saturated versions of "the body" and "knowing" for decades (see the first edition of *The Disability Studies Reader* edited by Lennard Davis in 1997), and more recently curriculum studies scholarship has questioned a sensorial hierarchy that privileges a visual portal, opening to consideration unique pathways to knowledge production and challenging the abjection and marginalization of "non-mainstream" onto-epistemologies (see Appelbaum, 2010; Gershon, 2011; Springgay, 2008). Psychologized teacher education research is largely a different story, however. It is difficult to find mainstream teacher education literature that would caution against the maximization of organized sensorial activation, that would *not* recommend "delivering" instruction through as many sensory portals simultaneously as possible, reinforcing the visual with the aural and the tactile, for example. In constructivist, learner centered pedagogies especially this kind of instructional design and sensory integration is highly valued as long as it does not inflame hyperactivity (Mills, 2016).

In his analysis of constructivist, learner centered approaches and teacher professional development, Tabulawa (2013) notes, however, that the reception of such movements in sub-Saharan African schools reveals its own lesson, indicating sharp differences in the cultural values that underpin teaching styles. While not directly interrogating the way in which a sensorium is positioned, Tabulawa delineates the onto-epistemolgoical assumptions that comport current trends in popular Western forms of instruction. What is promulgated by international aid agencies as relatively benign changes in instructional style, Tabulawa sees at best as forms of misunderstanding of cultural differences and contexts and at worse cultural domination by the west. Noting that movements such as constructivism were themselves well-intended critiques of the view of "ready-made," value-neutral facts being imparted to students as passive recipients, Tabulawa digs deeper to allude to the ways in which particular belief systems such as positivism and empiricism continue to operate through Western movements. Alternative approaches, like those offered through Progressive Education, may have been opposed to the excesses of previous styles, but may also have carried some of the same presumptions within them. Learner centered pedagogy is not for Tabulawa an innocuous or innocent, automatic good but that which emerged within particular spatiotemporal sites of production and it therefore carries specific cultural baggage and associations with it:

> Learner-centeredness has often been used interchangeably with "participatory", "democratic", "inquiry-based", "child/student-centered methods" and "discovery" methods. All these are strands of "Progressive Methods" whose origins can be traced to Jean-Jacques Rousseau and to the philosophical tradition of empiricism as propounded by the English philosopher John Locke. These strands differ in that they emphasise different degrees of learner autonomy.... There is general agreement that progressive methods are founded upon the social constructivist epistemology ... where knowledge is a product of social process and not solely an individual construct. Progressive Education views students as active participants in the learning process rather than as meek recipients of ready-made factual knowing in the teacher. (Tabulawa, 2013, pp. 3–4)

In asking why *learner centered* pedagogy, why in sub-Saharan Africa *now*, and why and how "tissue rejection" occurs in regard to implantation of a foreign organ, Tabulawa explains:

> The perceived utility of an innovation has implications for how it is received in its host environment. Teachers and students in the sub-Saharan context are mostly likely to evaluate the utility value of pedagogical innovation in terms of whether it is likely to enhance students' performance in tests and examinations, not in terms of whether it is likely to produce students with the character traits preferred in contemporary political life and the economy. Would teachers and students be ready to adopt and implement a pedagogy that has no apparent and immediate utility value to them? In the context of Africa, the answer is a clear "No". Thus, the very rationale for the learner-centered pedagogy might be its Achilles' heel. If the argument is admissible, then the pedagogy must be treated as problematic, instead of assuming, as the technicist approach does, that it is only technical issues to do with the innovation delivery system that matter. (Tabulawa, 2013, p. 18)

Like receptions of Rousseau's Émile which today can be positioned in technicist ways, minimizing the heated religious debates it participated in at publication, Tabulawa (2013) reminds the reader of the frames within which constructivist, learner centered pedagogy traveled. The conditions of possibility for such approaches to garner caché beyond their sites of production include for Tabulawa, the falling of the Berlin Wall in 1989, the subsequent move from a bipolar world order to a more unipolar world order, the heightened role of international funding agencies in sub-Saharan Africa that followed, the assumption that liberal democratization into a party political system offering "choice" is good, the belief that this should precede and then accompany reform into a capitalist economy, the assumption that such political and economic reform is aided through changing how schools teach, the assumption that changes in teaching style produce the attitudinal changes desired in students, the presumption that changes in teaching style improve students' test scores, and that only teaching styles that claim a kinship with democracy and choice can be associated with modernization, efficiency, and quality.

In a strange but potent twist, the turn-of-the-19th century phrenological texts published within Europe and the United States act as a kind of pivot in regard to the two above instances, exposing the politics of the senses in different directions. In looking "back" in time from the dates of Gallian publications, the discursive trajectories drawn upon reverse Rousseau's operationalization of the senses at a certain level, while in looking "forward," the role of "Africans" in developmental and international aid discourses that Tabulawa documents is clearly prefigured.

That is, what is striking in regard to the volatility around Émile's reception in the 1700s is that by the 1800s, a reversal had become possible: an appeal to the senses could be made to reinforce what was believed to be innate, not to undermine it. Scholars who might have concurred with Rousseau that the idea of Original sin in its Catholic form at least was suspect, could now also argue that there was something else inborn. Rather than being an evenly spread negative quality the "it" of the inborn was given an inherently graduated form across humans. The role attributed to the senses was not to overturn a belief in innateness but to reinforce it and to describe its gradient. Likewise, Gall's more frequent mention of "idiots" and "simpletons" compared to the sparser reference to "Africans" in his oeuvre still effects an ontological scale and a conflation. It puts "both" groups outside the high end of reason-morality, or what is labeled in much of his writing as "the moral and intellectual faculties," but it does so again on the basis of the role attributed to the senses, not just in the observed but in the one who presumes the right and entitlement to observe, classify, and publish. The following sections elaborate these reversals, intersections, and complexities, raising for broader consideration the stakes in ontological, epistemological, and onto-epistemological debates connected to education, the spatializing effects, and the risks of superficial appeal to the multisensory and multimodal as an automatic good.

PHRENOLOGY, PERCEPTION, AND SENSATION

> But when, by sensation, we understand only the impression of the external world on the senses, as most authors do, we neglect wholly the interior man

> and animals, and forget that the exterior world is known only so far as our interior has the faculty of perceiving it: and that, furthermore, this faculty is an abundant source of numerous sensations and ideas, by which each being preserves his individuality, consciousness and peculiar nature, though all are equally surrounded by the same objects. (Gall, 1835, p. 111)

Sensation is a vexed concept for Gall and one he turns on its head. Against much received opinion, he posits sensation as not just that which comes from an external environment but also from organs within the body. In *On the Origin of the Moral and Intellectual Faculties of Man, and the Conditions of Their Manifestation* (translated into English in 1835), Gall distinguishes between *perception*, as feelings about what is sensed, and *sensation*, the action on and from the organ or the portal. It also includes as part of sensation what today might be classified as beyond it, such as thinking:

> To taste, feel, see, hear, and touch, are sensations but we likewise feel pain and pleasure, itching, tickling, weariness, &c., produced by internal causes; we feel hunger, thirst, the calls of nature; we feel joy and sadness, hatred and love, humility and pride, hope and despair, desire, anguish, fear, terror, &c: the acts of our intellectual facilities, thinking, desiring, and wishing, are likewise sensations. (Gall, 1835, p. 111)

To this end, animals in addition to humans have a *consciousness* that perceptions and sensations inform, which Gall localizes to the nervous system and classifies as a faculty: "The faculty of awakening perceptions or sensation is common to the whole nervous system. To perceive and to feel are phenomena which we observe first and most generally in all beings endowed with the faculty of consciousness" (Gall, 1835, p. 111). What is crucial here is that consciousness is an a priori quality—it enables perceptions and sensations to be had at all and then consciousness is shaped by the specific qualitative content of those perceptions and sensations. Unlike some of his peers, Gall does not take the existence or shaping of consciousness to be driven mostly by or founded upon the operation of visual organs. The argument, however, requires the act of "observation" nonetheless, of "beings" such as plants, animals and humans to make its point. Ironically, then, while his argument about ontology is dependent upon acts of observation and of head squeezing (bumpology as it was satirically called), he treats the different senses with an equanimity that flattens a prior sensorial hierarchy which some of his peers preferred. He is at pains to point out that neither vision nor touch should be elevated and to this end he participates in a long history of debate in Western thought. The longer debate often conjoined questions over the nature of being to questions over *knowing* about being to questions over the *moral-intellectual* qualities that would enable one to know, as though one question naturally and deservedly led to the next in an unbroken sequence. In Gallian texts, the politics of knowledge is thus a "Western" affair, an obsession with ontology's relation to epistemology, within which the work that the senses can do and that education could effect is constrained by the presumptions of this sequence. He lands amid that sequencing upon a philosophy of *innatism* rationalized in psychophysiological form while leaving the door open for "powers" left relatively ambiguous, undefined and unspecified in terms of origin, a dilemma he arrives at in part through his analysis of the sensorium.

VISION, TOUCH, AND THE POLITICS OF KNOWLEDGE

It may seem that innatist theories are heavily challenged by supplication to a visual modality especially, for in a post-empiricist era if something is posited as innate within a conception of body as physical envelope, then one has to *show* that it is indeed "in there." How can a third party corroborate an innate quality, an inside "thing," that is not able to be gathered around and pointed to, drawn after human dissection, or later still, photographed? In the debates of the early 1800s over the politics of knowledge and configurations such as soul-mind-body relations, however, these are in a "sense" the wrong questions.

Phrenological research participated quite seriously and quite unevenly in an uncertain moment in which vision-as-visuality (the eye as a portal for viewing a thing in front of it) was under pressure for its role in truth production. Being able to "trick" someone into seeing something that others "knew" was not there (the acts of magicians, hypnotists, etc.) was available for street corner demonstration. The eyes could "see" that what people believed they "saw" was open to manipulation, setting in motion an infinite circularity. As such, the phrenological literature, weaving between village anecdotes, local demonstrations, and appeal to seemingly objective, outside observers and "fact," gives off a rather journalistic feel. It is born of the tussle between phenomenology and positivism, the first and the third person, and the uncertainty over the role attributed to the eyes in truth production, especially if humans could be "shown" to so easily be "tricked."

Discourses that invoke reference to terms associated today with vision are not, however, reducible to the operation of the human eye (Jay, 1994). Vision as revelation, vision as truth telling, or vision as seeing a picture demonstrates the broad range and uneven location of something that is now primarily coded as an ocular sense. As Levin (1997, p. 7) has noted, for example, references to vision have been and still are multitextual for "'visual perception' is never just a simple, immediate, straightforward, unproblematic presentation of the phenomenon of vision." Significantly, multitextuality points to a larger horizon of debate, tying discourses of vision to other positions where in question are "the formation of individual identity, the constitution of social relations, the cultural genealogy of stereotypes, the administrative power of the state, the visibility and accountability of governmental agents and agencies, the human relationship to nature and use of the environment, and the construction of discursive sites, of places and spaces, in the public sphere" (Levin, 1997, p. 7). The historicizing literature generally acknowledges this mulitextuality, following the Philosophy 101 arc—from ancient Greece to the 21st century West—pointing up shifting inscriptions of particular conceptual clusters and connected vocabularies including *being*, *light*, and *knowing* in different epistemes (Jay, 1994; Lechte, 2012) and it does so with sensitivity to vast differences in roles that discourses of vision have especially played in *claims to truth* (Tavares, 2016).

The difficulty this poses for reapproaching texts like Gallian ones are many. In *Genealogy and Ontology of the Image and Its Digital Future,* Lechte (2012) notes, for instance, that while in a digital world the presumption that "vision" is generally tied to "seeing," meaning a public consensus around what is commonsensically labeled as an image on a screen privileging observation through the eyes, in Plato's Greece anything that smacked of the status of an "image" was ranked a falsity. The "fact" that two people could claim to see an image at the same time did not make it Truth. Truth could not be anything but the original Forms, which in/famously could not be "seen" in the darkness of *The Republic's* cave. Reality was not the object you held in your hand or the picture of something on a wall, nor was reality the body. These "material things" were *illusions*, not "empirical evidence" or "data" in a qualitative study of a classroom. Truth and reality are understood to be elsewhere, away from material embodiment, and to be especially in the most ideal Form of all, the Form of the Good.

Here, vision is *not* reduced to human sight and the naked eye in "the observer" as Gall presumes. A human perceiver does not play a *foundational* role in which human consciousness does the noticing and selecting from a scene in front of the face. Moreover, physiological blindness is not the Other of vision. Such assumptions would naively gloss differences in cosmologies by casting modernist inscriptions back over a "subjectivity without subject" that has become almost impossible to relate to. Crucially, for Lechte, then, within a Platonic cosmology the human subject is not the driver of perception, nor necessarily distinguishable as "the subject" at all. Rather, how things come to notice remains ambiguous, the source is not necessarily singular and the location not necessarily in the head. In a world where "humans," gods, and animals mate, transmogrify, transact, and reincarnate vision becomes mentioned as an onto-epistemological strategy concerned with "proving" the moral superiority of Being over Becoming and pertains to the revelational apprehension of the Forms and the idealism of Goodness. It does not pertain to a route for truth production that travels unmediated through sensory portals aided by the brain (Baker, 2017).

> The impressions, whether they come from the external world through the senses, or from the internal by the general organs of sensations, must, then, be considered as indispensable conditions, without which no perception and no thought can take place. But, no impression from without, no irritation from within, can become a sensation or an idea, without the concurrence of the brain. The faculty of perceiving impressions, of retaining and comparing ideas, and making application of them, is by no means in proportion to the senses either in men or animals, as is proved by the example of idiots and simpletons. Thus, could we even have it demonstrated, that man, of all animals, has the most perfect senses, we should not thus obtain the explanation of his surpassing all others in intellectual faculties. (Gall, 1835, p. 128)

Phrenological scholarship, then, harkens back to Plato only in terms of the obsession with morality as the basis for answering questions over the nature of Becoming/Being and the essentialism attributed to kinds. The reduction of vision to *seeing with the eyes* moved along a different trajectory, often denoted back to faint beginnings in Aristotle's apparent scientism, moving forward in different incarnations from there (Baker, 2013). While Jay (1994) notes to some extent the differences between the Hellenic and Hebraic trajectories, and muddies the distinction between medieval ocularphobic and modern ocularcentric cultures, other literature moves beyond "the tyranny of Greece" and the Mideast (Bernal, 1987; Bynum, 1999). The role of what are now called the senses in epistemology, and especially the eyes, has been given a significantly longer lineage, going back at least to North African philosophies, particularly cosmologies circulating within ancient Egypt and Nubia, subsequently modified by Aristotle, whose preservation and reinterpretation as text is then attributed to Islamic scholars and Celtic monks, and thereby reintroduced into medieval Latin Europe where Aristotelianism flourishes among the Scholastics (Bynum, 1999; Clark, 2007).

This lineage, especially from Alhazen (10th century CE) onwards, marks the messy beginnings of optics, where *vision-as-visuality* starts to emerge as a stronger part of the rationale for truth production and as a conduit of proof. A more ocularcentric belief system takes hold beyond the theatricalization of Christian doctrine and adoration of ornaments (Jay, 1994, p. 39). Such a belief system in Byzantine and medieval cultures becomes presumed *and* augmented later in the study of "species" to which Gall repeatedly refers in naturalizing ways (Jay, 1994; Lechte, 2012). The modern inflection of ocularcentrism in what Jay (1994, p. 3) separates out as theology and science enables elaboration of "exosomatic organs" called technology —the effort to extend, substitute or enhance the limited power of the eye. This included drawings of dissected corpses in anatomical texts as a practice of "scientific representation" that scholars such as Gall participated in and were praised for advancing (Richardson, 2001).

Optics is the belief system most associated today with ocularcentrism in an objectivist sense: seeing through the eyes is believing, knowing *must* come through (the now) five senses but especially important are the eyes, and "to show is to know" becomes a key condition of proof. As noted above, though, by the late 1800s confidence in the objectivity of what came through the eyes had waned, meaning a new role for the eyes in truth production had to be found. If we could not agree upon what we saw, or if what one saw was invisible to others, then how would truth be reached through Cartesian appeals to *method* and a subject/object distinction?

Gall's position on the play of the senses both participates in this history of debate over multitextual links between discourses of vision, truth production and being and at the same time departs from some of its major presuppositions. He allocates the senses only a shaping role in regard to what is already posited as innate and describes the brain as a series of organs that are intermediary. His position on vision-as-visuality assumes blindness as Other but does not automatically connect seeing or blindness to "bad" or "good" in simplistic ways, insofar as he asserts that the best painters are not the best painters because of their eyes, but because of their inherent faculties, their *mind*, not their *eyesight*. This means that the best painters do not necessarily have the most acuity in their visual organs, just as he notes the best musicians are sometimes deaf.

He matches this "disconnect" between a refined sensory portal and a displayed talent to his conclusion about touch: those with the most acutely perceptive or sensitive apparatuses do not necessarily make the most intelligent and inventive animals or humans. Whereas today in many settings to withhold an infant (within developmental psychology's construction of ability) from playing with a host of toys and common objects, from feeling and manipulating their shape and banging them together, from pulling apart and pushing along the floor, would be considered tantamount to deprivation, for Gall, better order in thought is not reducible to that which comes to us as via sensations such as touch. Engaging with objects and others does matter but only because of reciprocity with the existing inner faculties. Touch especially is not the great distinguisher or a superior, foundational or integrative sense:

> But, are the ideas acquired by means of touch, sufficient of themselves, to establish better order in thought? Can they rectify the errors of the mind, give birth to industry, to the arts, and invention? Is the degree of perfection

> of the nature of animals a consequence of greater delicacy of touch? Are our intellectual faculties and those of animals, as much more numerous, as the organs of touch are more in number, and more delicate? Does a more perfect touch afford more precise and more extended knowledge. And do animals choose things proper to their preservation, with so much the more certainty as their organs of touch are more supple? Can touch produce attention, memory, judgment, imagination, abstract ideas, curiosity, desire of instruction, the appetites, and the passions? Can we regard it as the first origin of all these faculties? or, must we rather consider it as an instrument, as a means, which have been created for the service of faculties of a superior order, and put in reciprocal relation with them? (Gall, 1835, p. 120)

The set up enables Gall to conclude that something else must operate to differentiate beings:

> Thus have I demonstrated, that it does not belong to the touch alone, to give us a knowledge of the world without us that sensations take place, not only by; means of the external senses, but likewise in the interior of the organization that we cannot call the touch, the corrector of the other senses that the hands, when; there exists no faculty of a superior order, cannot invent that the whole use of the touch is either arts or tools limited to procuring the ideas of distance, extent, form, rest, motion, moisture and dryness, and the degree of solidity of objects; that, in other respects, it must be regarded as the instrument of the superior faculties, these superior faculties, such as the inclinations, propensities, different modes of industry, and the faculties, cannot be determined, conjectured, or explained by the organs of touch. We are, then, obliged to seek other organic conditions, as the causes of all the faculties which we cannot derive from this sense. (Gall, 1835, pp. 126–127)

The "other organic conditions" that must explain the difference can be understood as a *faculty*, a faculty which sometimes blurs mind and brain into being one unit and sometimes includes mention of soul, too. Faculty here meant inborn, and it was via patho-anatomy that the locus for genuine differentiation was believed to be revealed: "The functions of the mind are deranged by the lesion of the brain: they are not immediately deranged by the lesion of other parts of the body" (Gall, 1798, p. 311). The brain draws its role as intermediary and as important via the logic integral to German enlightenment theories of expression. Such theories posited that internal essences attain their manifestation as external phenomena (Hoff, 1992). This creates a sequence of *invisible essence/first cause—instinct/faculty/power/function—organ—behaviour*, which is the sequence through which certainty was reinscribed into judgments, linking claims about innate qualities to "evidence" of phenotype and behaviour. The analyst or researcher appears to start at the end of the sequence with the observations and squeezing that then suggest the existence (or otherwise) of qualities and their first cause, working their way back.

Gallian texts thus generally attempt to offer a correction to the overestimation of the role of the senses in this "working back" and especially in those who oppose innatism and attribute talents to an exterior influence. As the examples of vision-as-visuality and touch underscore, the volumes of his major work are staged to eradicate any "exterior" environmental influence from accounting for the *origin* of behavior. To this end, unlike Rousseau who, while attributing "something" to an interior domain permitted the senses to make the selfish Will of a child into a collective *moi against* its inclination, Gall more heavily aligns the operation of the senses with shaping what is already given inside, *a trellis to a fundament, neither an implanting of entirely new material, nor a complete redirection*. This formula in turn constrains the definition and role of education around a very particular version of determinism tied to the emergence of a modern episteme. Here, a scopic regime is forming that separates and then tries to link back together "things" and "words," the to and fro motoring claims to truth. This plays out, for instance, in how Gall elevates the organs of the brain—their shape, lumps and bumps—as a visual and haptic slate (thing) and how systems of language are referred to (as words and signs) to prove that the senses cannot be the *origin* of the moral and intellectual faculties that set humans apart from both animals and each other.

LINKING SENSATION TO DETERMINISM AND THE POSSIBILITIES AND LIMITS OF EDUCATION

> Whence come the words which do not precisely designate determinate ideas, but simply the mode of thinking; the prepositions, conjunctions, interjections, adverbs of interrogation and exclamation.... Do not the deaf and dumb, who possess reason, but who are deprived of the faculty of expressing themselves by articulate language, depict their internal sensations by gestures, which absolutely have nothing in common with the external world? (Gall, 1835, p. 130)

For Gall, those who attribute Man's nature and behavior primarily to external, exterior, or environmental influence try to have it both ways:

> This uniformity is, consequently, the strongest proof that nothing can derange the plan, which nature has prescribed by means of organization. For the rest, these panegyrists of the creative power of education, are in direct contradiction with themselves. At one time, the uniformity observed among men, serves to prove that education does everything; at another, in order to explain the difference in characters, they allege the impossibility of the greater part of individuals receiving a uniform education. (Gall, 1835, p. 149)

This does not mean that education should not be engaged in, however, for the influence of it in shaping the disposition makes the difference between "savage" and not. The child with not too little energy and not too much is the best recipient of instruction and in terms of innateness there is no difference between the theory as applied to "genius" and "idiot."

> genius is only the energetic activity of some quality or some faculty. If, then, in cases where the faculties have the greatest energy, the cause which produces it, and which is most striking, is inherent in the organization, we must naturally conclude that the cause of their ordinary activity is equally founded in the organization. Difference of more and less proves nothing against the common origin of obscure and decided faculties. (Gall, 1835, p. 144)

While decided faculties do not always need formal instruction (for Gall, to become great like Mozart or evil like Nero required no instruction) animals as for humans are recipients of a certain inborn power, defining *education-as-instruction*, like teacher centered pedagogy, as that which guides, not that which can implant or totally redirect.

> Neither man nor animals have any limb, any instrument, in order to use it, but they use them because they have them.... We must then admit, that each animal, in consequence of its organization, has received, from nature ingenious aptitudes, instincts, propensities, proper determinate talents, and that the power of things external, of instruction and education, is limited to giving it more or less modification. The hypothesis of the tabula rasa, and of the creative power of education, is it more admissible for the human race? (Gall, 1835, p. 138)

This version of determinism, as the opening quote to this chapter also underscores, does not follow a standard structural-functional logic. We do not have limbs because we need to use them, to survive or to evolve. Rather, the reverse: we have limbs that we then find uses for, which can in turn lead to survival and evolution – or not. This subtle displacement of a Creator designing limbs for humans as evidence of some kind of organic, sensorial superiority relocates the place of education pragmatically within the domain of the invisible play of "powers." The superior faculty of mind or soul-mind of the (non-savage, non-idiot) human for Gall helps humans to make more of the environment, to make different things of sensation from the person next to you, and of one's inherent dispositions.

MATERIALITY AS "PROOF" OF "KIND" OR "KIND" AS "PROOF" OF MATERIALITY?

> The degree of address, industry, and intelligence, with which an animal is endowed, has not for its principle his trunk, or his tail, which serves him

> for a trowel man does not invent because he has hands but the; animal and the man have these organs, because their internal organization is endowed with the faculties which are in relation with these. Certain organs may be indispensable to execute certain things yet we cannot; attribute to them the thought, which leads to constructing a nest or a hut; to the invention of printing, or weaving. (Gall, 1835, p. 124)

What is significant in phrenology more broadly and in Gallian texts specifically is how the description of an organ operates in tandem *with a particular definition of the material*—the material-as-*organization*—and with the delimitation of education to *education-as-instruction*. Gall argues that there is a period after birth *in which no instruction has been seen* but in which behaviors of newborns occur and this claim buttresses the view of innateness. It combines with how the seemingly neutral passage of time into adulthood can only pass to reveal the innate, a movement over which one has little control.

> Might I not ask whence the first men, who were surrounded only by beasts, obtained their faculties, and how they created or invented them? Even at the present time, are not many men, in their infancy, more surrounded by animals than by men? Why do not these children receive the instincts and propensities of animals as well as the faculties of man? If children had not the same dispositions as their parents and instructors, how could they be capable of receiving their instruction and profiting by their example? In the first years, when children are almost solely in the hands of their mothers, of nurses, and of women, boys always distinguish themselves from girls, and one child is perfectly distinct from another. After this period nothing can give rise to a resemblance between the faculties of the man and the woman, nor between those of different individuals. In fine, do we know any art by which an instructor can create in children envy, love, attachment, anger, goodness or wickedness, ambition, pride, &c.? Do we know how to create any talent? This power so little belongs to man, that even when we are our own absolute masters, we cannot escape the changes which the succession of years produces in our moral and intellectual faculties. Every thing confirms the truth of what Herder says, that education cannot take place except by imitation, and consequently by the passage from the original to the copy. (Gall, 1835, p. 139)

The differential manifestation is not proof of lack of innateness but its intricate operation: "in certain individuals, some organs remain always in arrear, while others acquire the greatest energy. But this explanation shows again, that all the moral qualities and intellectual faculties are innate" (Gall, 1835, p. 145). The definition of material-as-organization becomes all-consuming here, allowing no quality outside of its purview.

The definition of material-as-organization is expanded to refer also to function. Together, *the organization and the function* provide the "evidentiary base" or condition of proof for why certain beings act in one way and not another.

> All which we have said proves, that man and animals do not perform what they execute, by means of touch, because they have this sense more or less perfect, but that it is necessary to admit, that the external organs, the senses, are calculated to adapt themselves to the internal faculties. Would there not exist a perpetual contradiction between the propensities, the faculties, and and would not the internal faculties be rendered useless by the impotence of the external organs, if these were not fitted to execute what the internal ones command? Give to the tiger, bathed in blood, the feet and the teeth of the sheep, and to the sheep, the claws and murderous teeth of the lion, and instantly, by this contradictory arrangement of apparatuses, you destroy the existence of these two animals. (Gall, 1835, p. 123)

This is not a neutral horizon, however. There are some qualities or faculties a "society" prefers over others, some kinds of being preferred over others. For instance, in arguing *against* the idea that the play of the senses makes the mental difference between men and animals, Gall offers a correction, by way of "savage nations" and the "man of genius":

> this mode of expression [of attributing everything to an exterior environment] again supposes the error, that man has senses more perfect than animals; and, as, on the other hand, we generally attribute to savage nations the most delicate senses, it would be from them that we ought to expect the most profound philosophy and the feeblest instinct; which will hardly be admitted. (Gall, 1835, p. 131)

And

> The greatest men, it is true, bear the impress of their age, and cannot entirely defend themselves from the impression of the objects which surround them still, we constantly see, that he who possesses a dominant energetic quality or faculty, pursues his route, and seizes with force the object which nature has pointed out to him. Thomas, in writing the eulogy of Descartes, did well not to dwell much upon his education. "For," said he, "when the question relates to extraordinary men, we have to consider education much less than nature. There is an education for common men; the man of genius has the education which he gives himself, and which consists principally in destroying and effacing, that which he has received." ... "Neither does good education make the great character, nor does bad education destroy it. Heroes, of all classes, come ready formed from the hands of nature, and with uncontrollable qualities." (Gall, 1835, p. 143)

Together, the automatic references to "savages" and "idiots" create a potent conflated force for placing the gradient of innateness within materiality. "Savagery" was repetitively judged in the era by skin color and location such as continent. "Idiocy" and "simpletons" were judged via a fear of asymmetry and expressions taken as ramblings. *Materiality-as-organization-and-function* shores up the ontological spatialization *already available* in demographic reasonings, attributing it to organs. Materiality operates as the intermediary between science and religion, between potential Designer and designed. It conjoins the classificatory regimes common to European high colonialism of the time that linked savage and civil, idiot and sane, as poles on a spectrum of worth. Rather than suggesting no hope for education-as-instruction, however, phrenological reasoning circumscribes what education is and what it can achieve in particular forms, circularly related to the definition of the material:

> The builder-wasp has already learned, while yet a larva, the masonry of his mother; the bird learns from those who have given him life, to build his nest, to sing, to migrate...; and man would not become man, would remain a savage and idiot, without the means furnished by education. (Gall, 1835, p. 137)

Here, what emerges is a pivotal series of assumptions with which the field of education is still grappling and to which Tabulawa (2013) draws our attention in terms of what comes to sub-Saharan Africa as recommendations for innovation. In order to overturn a conservative Catholic view of Original sin, Rousseau gives air to the sensorium. In order to reinstate a notion of the inborn and to differentiate it as either a talent or a criminality—what is innate could be "good" *or* "bad"—Gall gives the senses an adumbrated role, a role in *shaping* or unleashing, but not in *founding*, the powers/faculties/instincts/capacities called mind. Western theories of education tend today to vacillate between variations of these two possibilities, appealing to genetics or environment or an interplay—from reinvigorations of the bell curve to calls for social justice and attention to cultural contexts. What remains in play, however, and perhaps inadvertently, is belief in the connection between *being*, *knowing*, the *moral-intellectual* and *differentiation*—the sequence that sets the parameters for a sensorium to matter *as matter* in a particular form. In the final section then, I briefly contrast this sequence to debates over roles of the sensorium and especially the eyes in Buddhist archives. Here, while coming close to Gall's notion of the distinction between a fleshy, sensory portal and the "power" that must innervate the organ's ability to act in a particular way (its special sense-power), Buddhist debates, which also trade on an ontological hierarchy, do not play out their soteriological project within a conception of the sensorium as that which ought to be *always* activated, *always* already involved, at least where ultimate Truth is concerned.

BEYOND NATURAL AND SUPERNATURAL SENSES

Perhaps in part because of the pictoral, visual, and contemplative turns more broadly across academic fields, reference to Buddhist theories of seeing and visuality appear repetitively in the Anglophone debates now referred to as Western Buddhisms or Buddhist epistemologies. And just as there was considerable discursive space for Gall to differ from his peers in regard to the role of the senses, so in Buddhist archives the debate is wide-ranging and plural. While it is impossible to summarize centuries of commentatorial tradition in any archive it is especially so in Buddhist archives where scholar-meditator traditions move from oral to written to the beyond written and beyond visual. Lukicheva, Suter, and Behr (2016) note the impossibility and the complexity that includes and exceeds technical translation issues. They question where one would even draw the line around Buddhist archives, and by extension, one could include the lines around "Eastern" or "Western" in 21st century debates. They note, for instance, in their recent call for a "Vision and Visuality in Buddhism and Beyond" workshop that it is not just that interpretive and etymological issues are many but that "References to Buddhist theories of perception and visuality, their specific terminologies and metaphorical vocabulary, are recurrent throughout epistemological and aesthetic reflections in East Asia. This is true even for texts that do not explicitly relate to a Buddhist context" (Lukicheva, Suter, & Behr, 2016, p. 1).

Hatchell's (2013a, 2013b) work is significant and the focus here, then, because it delves deftly into and across Buddhist archives (especially through links to broader Indian philosophies that preceded Buddhism) in ways that are sensitive to such issues and to the irreducibility of differences between Western philosophical and biological constructs around discourses of vision. Hatchell posits that Buddhist literature contains a number of interrelated discussions of seeing but that seeing and vision are not exclusively reference to the biological eye. The discussions are engaged in by "particular Buddhists in particular times and places [who] have offered their own answers, and those collectively can be read as an extended discussion about seeing that moves across many of the Buddhist disciplines: epistemology, ethics, physiology, ritual, cosmology, myth, poetry, visual arts, and yogic practice. Each of these fields is, in turn, informed by Buddhists' distinctive ideas about the visual faculties" (Hatchell, 2013, p. 340). The Buddhist discussions thus draw multitextually upon a variety of traditions that investigate the act of seeing, meditative practices of looking and visualization, the ritual use of visual arts, and literary metaphorical references to light. With this breadth and diversity in mind, Hatchell identifies a basic typology of Buddhist "eyes" (he suspends the term) along four trajectories, including (1) the function of the ordinary eyes, (2) ethical dimensions of the eyes, (3) the attainment of supernatural eyes, and (4) types of eyes that are involved in Buddhist soteriology (Hatchell, 2013, p. 339). Such a typology, rather than aiming to reduce rich commentatorial traditions operates "with the broader goal of providing a set of ideas that will be useful in thinking about Buddhist perspectives on seeing and the visual world" (p. 340).

Relative to how Gall positions the role of the senses in the sequence for differentiating types of being—the senses can only shape an origin or foundation that is already there and this results in the marks accounted for or categorized as differences, such as species or talents—the turn to various discourses of "the eye" and of "seeing" have different philosophical starting points and roles in Buddhist archives. Starting points can include illustrating the distinction between everyday perceptions (defined as *contact* between the organ, the sense-power within it, the object perceived in front of it, plus the feeling it arouses) and Ultimate Truth, which is not beholden to the illusion of perception/contact, to words or things. Starting points are not that of monotheism or monism, then, but are soteriological, related to the alleviation of suffering and the end of cyclical existence. Invoking discourses of the eye therefore requires attention to which version of the eye, how the relationship formed between seeing and illusion causes suffering, and how that can be reformed into a non-seeing/beyond-seeing, non-conceptuality that has no essential content yet is Real—emptiness.

Attention to ordinary or biological eyes, for instance, is given across texts in ways that position such eyes as both useful in the pragmatic navigation of daily life and as that which is to be withheld where higher awareness is concerned. The relationship described between ordinary eyes and perception is for illustrating everyday reality/perception as illusion (illustration, as though a finite and fixed arbiter, is also an illusion, however). Perception of "objects" as though they have distinct essences that make them different from each other leads to attachment, grasping, and holding on because contact involves "feeling" and in this form points to entrapment in cyclic existence and karmic rebirth. The upshot initially is that the rope lying on the floor in the dark, mistaken for a snake and feared accordingly, is no more Real than the snake —both rope and snake are illusions and both generated feelings. Beyond ordinary or biological eyes are appeals to supernatural eyes that exceed what mainstream Western optics can cope with: seeing that can occur in light or dark, when eyes are open or closed in the biological form, seeing as being able to discern someone's karmic past, seeing into someone's future rebirth, and so forth. This "talent" which is arguably how Gall might have classified such "demonstrations" is not for ego or showing off as a party trick, but a series of "capacities" nonetheless that can be either cultivated or inborn. Supernatural eyes are but a stage, though, on the way to a greater Buddha vision where eyes become the metaphor (but biological eyes are not what is being referred to as the meaning of "eyes" here) and where what might be classified as extrasensory or supernatural in psychology is not that remarkable either. Buddhist soteriology requires the "path of seeing" to be understood as transcendent or non-conceptual knowing. While forms (color and shape) are experienced visually with the biological eyes Buddha-realization is not just about seeing through or beyond color and shape but both much more and much less. Matter-as-organization-and-function per Gallian formulation is less the mediator of knowledge here and more the indicator of a trap within which "words" and "things" participate to continuously fuel attachments. That is, appealing to concepts or objects as proof, or intellectualizing and theorizing the relationship between them, are part of the same cycle of attachment, keeping one focused on and pinned into the illusion of essential differences. "Concepts," for instance, are no better than "objects" in that regard. Concepts are formed out of the apparently distinct threads that become grouped together and named as a subject or object (like "people" or "pots") (Hathcell, 2013a). In the end, this naming and analytical process is just another illusion distracting from the realization of emptiness, of non-spatialization between "non"-things. The question remains, however, why use discourses of the eye as the pedagogical tool to get to such soteriological endpoints? For Hatchell, in Buddhist literature the,

> common turn to seeing is simply that visual experience is so fundamental and so visceral that a critique of substantiality has more effect than, for instance, a critique of a pot. If the project of emptiness is designed to shock the reader out of closely held assumptions, purely theoretical or intellectual approaches might be less effective than deconstructions of something so precious as the visual capacity. In this way.... Buddhists use the topic of seeing for the contrast it provides with intellectual or conceptual activity, or as a way to demonstrate how the process of knowing can happen in the absence of any reified act—how there is no "seeing," but yet we can still see. (Hatchell, 2013a, p. 345)

Gall's version of complexity, in which he does not elevate seeing or touch over other senses, but in which he does need observation of ducks, animals, humans, and so forth, and the feeling of heads, bumps and lumps to make his point, is dedicated to answering a relatively simple question: why are his school peers different from each other? Based on the answer that he gives, what can education be, and not be? Discussions about seeing in Buddhist archives offer a "different" version of complexity and simplicity. They turn to such key issues as discourses of vision and kinds of eyes because they are thought involved in human suffering and transcendence from it (Hatchell, 2013a, p. 346). The debate over the distinction between inborn and environment which preoccupied Gall operate in Buddhist archives upon a a broader horizon of the wheel of karma, but the reference to karma is but one part of a much wider cosmology that exceeds planet earth and that includes the ability to see between what today might be called galaxies, parallel universes, other worlds not currently available to the perception of most humans. More than that, this kind of hyper-attuned seeing is not necessarily defined as extraordinary or freakish, but as a step on a pathway to something even more integrated. Thus, when ordinary biological eyes are something to be wary of and the visual faculties are to be treated at the everyday level as things to be cast downward, restrained or transcended it is not the same move or analytical process, frame, or horizon as Gall's relationship to sight. Moreover, looking "more fully at Buddhist varieties of otherworldly eyes and its positive treatment of vision, it becomes clear that they [Buddhist texts] are interested in more than 'non-seeing'" (Hatchell, 2013a, p. 346). For Gall, you can never escape what you are born but how it unfolds may vary a bit and the variety is to be understood as both tethered and good. It is good that a duck is not an eagle—it keeps nature interesting—and it is good that man's mind makes him more intelligent than an eagle. It is bad when what unfolds is criminality, savagery, idiocy, and so forth. In Buddhist soteriology, the claim that one cannot escape what one is born is untrue. And significantly, the "proof" of this is not an organ or series of organs called brain, nor a substance called matter, nor a science of facts, but simply the existence of "beings" who non-conceptually "know" that "beings" are able to be enlightened and who find it very difficult to explain what that is like because to do so, the explaining, risks giving reinforcement to the very tools, attachments and feelings that constitute an obstacle (albeit one that can be overcome) within the initial steps on a pathway to enlightenment.

The provincialism within Buddhist archives, the belief in ontological hierarchy and elevation of a small number of beings as free from karmic cycles, makes the sense-power of sight easy to use for instructive purposes but ultimately unnecessary—one does not need everyday eyesight or any other "sense" to be continuously activated in order to learn, to evacuate, or to achieve awareness such as "Buddha eyes" and Samādhi. In contrast, the provincialism in Gallian texts is that visual acuity is considered unnecessary to become a great painter but is necessary to construct an argument around psychophysiology. Without privileging observation of behavior posited as visible, exterior, and in motion Gall cannot make the claim that "no instruction" has been given immediately after birth in certain species. Because he reduces education to instruction imparted by another and because he could not "see" instruction in certain scenarios, he believes education has not occurred at that point. So, a newborn, like a duckling walking straight to the water without a visible lesson by a parent, is classified as *knowing* what to do and thereby must be relying on something innate. Education here becomes direct instruction only and must have a clearly visible sender and receiver. Unlike Buddhist archives, Gallian texts do not depict this production of a narrative as an example of an *illusion* illustrated with colorful details. Rather in Gallian texts, and this is crucial, the role of the senses and the philosophical assumptions turn the duck walking to the water into a "fact" that bespeaks determinism in its silence and that illustrates for Gall an organic, innate foundation and origin for "difference."

CONCLUSION

The mocking that accompanied and exceeded Gall's work has obscured to some extent the impact that psychophysiology generated in many fields. Typically, the historical literature on phrenology points to such innovations as the belief in cerebral localization, the contributions his detailed human anatomical dissections provided, opening different angles on the relationship between brain and spine, and the shift from metaphysical to biological conceptions of mind and behavior. The analysis here has suggested that the latter especially is not so cut and dried, that the paradoxes, complexity and simplicity of what traveled through Gallian rationalizations relies heavily on ill-defined "powers" whose origin sometimes references a Creator and the divine directly, sometimes displaces the existence of such a concept or figure, and sometimes buries the metaphysical ghost in the biological machine.

The upshots of this mélange of positions are too many to summarize here. Important to recognize, however, is that the extension of the Gallian construction of innateness and origin has been both disastrous and obvious. Across the 1800s, public schools are invented, implemented for some groups and withheld from others, villages and cities become nations at a more rapid pace, citizenship for some groups and not others, and eugenics emerges as a powerful globalizing discourse, the right to live and reproduce for some groups and not others. This chapter has not argued that Gallian texts are somehow solely responsible for such divisions and hatreds, nor that there is any single starting point for societies moving from sovereignty and monarchy to disciplinary and institutional authority. Rather, it has identified one of the trajectories and one of the moments in which long-held beliefs about demography and ontological gradients were converted in a messy and inconsistent way from "the spiritual" to "the material," from prior, confident and straight out references to belief in an exteriorized Creator to descriptions of ill-defined "powers" in a human interior. The analysis here has not posited that this is a complete and utter substitution or totalization. It has demonstrated instead the role that a sensorium has played in the mediation, in the restriction of interest to an organological locus, in contradistinction to other possibilities such as Platonic cosmology and Buddhist archives.

This task is made all the more difficult and seemingly self-implicative because claiming "differences" or "distinction" is part of the topic, problems and methods here revisited. For this reason, this chapter has not claimed to occupy some pure position of an "outside" or emanate from a non-conceptual knowledge. Rather, it has illustrated how a moral-intellectual high ground, which critiques of "Contradiction!" leveled through social justice discourses frequently assume, becomes positioned as a zone and a capacity. For Rousseau, being able to name religion as a problem meant something else had become available in "worldviews" that would make a system of beliefs appear as a formal religion rather than something else. Religion could no longer just operate unspoken as way of life in the background and foreground of how things get done in an area. Rather than position religion as absolutely everything, in which case "religion" and "moral-intellectual" would not need to be named as separate at all, Rousseau advocated a form of pedagogy that would not teach formal religion until near adulthood, and then fled for his life. By the time of Gall, referring to the moral-intellectual as a *faculty/capacity/power*, makes it an "it," a zone within a wider, lateral discourse and an interior force within a deeper, vertical discourse. The "it" of faculty/capacity/power is relocated, displaced from the Biblical narrative of Original sin into an organic home that has a gradient to it. The appeal to gradient is used to explain how differences attributed to beings such as species and between humans can be based on mind's relationship to brain and sometimes soul.

In retrospect, such discursive moves act as a bridge to the later genetic determinism that would undergird the Stanford-Binet IQ tests of the early twentieth century and later the bell curve in the United States (Baker, 2005), the latter of which seemed particularly invested in positioning African American students especially as though behind all other U.S. populations—a worldview dedicated to sustaining deep prejudice via decontextualized demographic reasonings, repeatedly debunked as racist and mismeasure (Chase, 1977; Gould, 1981). In earlier Gallian texts, the stage for such debates in written form is already set. The role of the sensorium in all its richness was called upon to reinforce and re-justify a spatializing effect within an essentialist version of Life and to try (unsuccessfully) to install a firm line between epistemology as subject matter content and ontology as a kind of predetermined being. This being could be guided by epistemology but never totally redirected, resecuring prior hierarchies amid what Alain de Botton (2005) might call "status anxiety." In trying to separate ontology from epistemology, education as direct instruction becomes the only kind. The mother duck has not been seen directly teaching the duckling to walk to the water, therefore no instruction or learning is believed to have occurred and the behavior is thereby described as instinctive and innate.

The chapter has also indicated how one major role of the multimodal and multisensory in constructivist-inspired pedagogies was to challenge such monoculturalism and innatism, to augment the view of non-neutrality of "bare facts," to affirm that there are multiple learning styles, preferences, and funds of knowledge, and to offer a more democratic flatness between who and what, teacher and learner, making less certain any claim to universal truth. Such orientations helped to some extent to blur ontology and epistemology into onto-epistemology in a chicken/egg like fashion in which education becomes redefined as a moving target and open journey, rather than static, unitized, prefigured, and objectives-driven.

One of the coins that link such apparently binary approaches to education—Gallian notions of education as teacher centered direct instruction for innatist qualities relative to constructivist, learner centered pedagogy—is the faith in the material-empirical-sensory as condition of proof and as that which makes augmentation and unfoldment of character possible. It is little wonder, then, that more than 100 years after the phrenological movement and debates over the sensorium as they connect to education, Tabulawa (2013) sees in constructivist, learner centered approaches less a radical progressive education and more of the same positioning of "Africans" as subjects-objects of reform indebted to philosophies of matter, to positivism and empiricism as dominating the politics of knowledge, as conditions of proof about kinds and being. This may raise within teacher education and curriculum studies an uncomfortable realization—the contemporary elevated appeal to matter and sensation may be considered dangerous in contexts both "at home" and "abroad."

The chapter has also underscored not simply the flashpoints and dangers inherent in phrenological discourses indebted to particular assumptions about the nature of reality, but also the limits of those assumptions' reach and the restriction in their fundament. In Platonic revelationalism and Buddhist archives, appeals to matter in whatever form do not secure proof or verification at the end of a system of reasoning or during a process of argumentation. Nor do they settle or resolve battles over "cultural differences" or "clashes in worldviews." Appeals to matter and subjects-objects with perceived innate essences that are presumed to be different are recognized more as a starting point for deconstruction, keyed to a less highly valued everyday perception that indexes the illusion that can be dispelled, in different ways and for different reasons in "each" case. The questions that this intersection of genealogical trajectories and transphilosphical traces leave for teacher education and curriculum studies are, then, many and profound. While the multifarious directions this analysis suggests cannot be raised singly within the space here, one of the most generative is also perhaps one of the most simple "What do educators think is being proven or achieved by appeal to a sensorium?"

NOTES

1. I have mapped the breadth of associations that the term discourses of vision incorporates in Baker (2017).
2. There is voluminous comparative literature on "Eastern" and "Western" religion and the same for Buddhism. In regard to the latter, Lopez (2012), McMahan (2008), and Sharf (2015) offer less simplistic introductions to issues beyond the linguistic and terminological, within and outside Asian contexts.

REFERENCES

Appelbaum, P. (2010). Against sense and representation: Researchers as undetectives. *Educational Insights, 14*(1), 1–25.

Baker, B. (2017). To show is to know? Conceptions of evidence and discourses of vision in social science and education research. *Curriculum Inquiry, 47*(2), 151–174.

Baker, B. (2013). *William James, sciences of mind, and anti-imperial discourse*. New York, NY: Cambridge University Press.

Baker, B. (2005). From the genius of the man to the man of genius. Part two: Inheriting (ideas about) genius. *History of Education Review, 34*(2), 78–94.

Baker, B. (2001a). *In perpetual motion: Theories of power, educational history, and the child*. New York, NY: Peter Lang.

Baker, B. (2001b). (Ap)Pointing the canon: Rousseau's Émile, visions of the state, and education. *Educational Theory, 51*(1), 1–41.

Bernal, M. (1987). *Black Athena: The Afroasiatic roots of classical civilization*. New Brunswick, NJ: Rutgers University Press.

Bynum, E. B. (1999). *The African unconscious: Roots of ancient mysticism and modern psychology (Counseling and Development Series)*. New York, NY: Teachers College Press.

Chase, A. (1977). *The legacy of malthus: The social costs of the new scientific racism*. New York, NY: Knopf; Random House.

Clark, S. (2007). *Vanities of the eye: Vision in early modern European culture*. Oxford, England: Oxford University Press.

De Botton, A. (2005). *Status anxiety*. New York, NY: Vintage International.

Gould, S. J. (1981). *The mismeasure of man*. New York, NY: W. W. Norton and Company.

Gall, F. J. (1798). Letter from Dr. F. J. Gall to Joseph Freiherr von Retzer, upon the functions of the brain, in man and animals. *Der Neue Teutsche Merkur, 3*, 311–332. doi:www.historyofphrenology.org.uk/texts/retzer.htm

Gall, F. J. (1835). *On the functions of the brain and each of its parts with observations on the possibility of determining the instincts, propensities, and talents, or the moral and intellectual dispositions of men and animals, by the configuration of the brain and head. Vol. 1: On the origin of the moral and intellectual faculties of man, and the conditions of their manifestation*. Boston, MA: Marsh, Capen & Lyon.

Gershon, W. (2011). Embodied knowledge: Sounds as educational systems. *Journal of Curriculum Theorizing, 27*(2), 66–81.

Hatchell, C. (2013a). Buddhist visual worlds I: The eyes and ways of seeing. *Religion Compass, 7*(9), 339–348.

Hatchell, C. (2013b). Buddhist visual worlds II: Practices of visualization and vision. *Religion Compass, 7*(9), 349–360.

Hoff, T. L. (1992). Gall's psychophysiological concept of function: The rise and decline of "internal essence". *Brain and Cognition, 20*(2), 378–398.

Jay, M. (1994). *Downcast eyes: The denigration of vision in twentieth-century French thought*. Berkeley, CA: University of California Press.

Lechte, J. (2012). *Genealogy and ontology of the Western image and its digital future*. New York, NY: Routledge.

Levin, D. M. (Ed.). (1997). *Sites of vision: The discursive construction of sight in the history of philosophy*. Cambridge, MA: MIT Press.

Lopez, D. S. Jr (2012). *The scientific Buddha: His short and happy life* (The Terry Lectures Series). New Haven, CT: Yale University Press.

Lukicheva, P., Suter, R., & Behr, W. (2016). Vision and visuality in Buddhism and beyond Retrieved July 5, 2017, from https://www.academia.edu/31198640/_with_Polina_Lukicheva_Rafael_Suter_Vision_and_Visuality_in_Buddhism_and_Beyond

Mills, K. A. (2016). *Literacy theories for the digital age: Social, critical, multimodal, spatial, material and sensory lenses*. Bristol, England: Multilingual Matters.

Davis, L. J. (Ed.). (1997). *The disability studies reader*. New York, NY: Routledge.

McMahan, D. L. (2008). *The making of Buddhist modernism*. New York, NY: Oxford University Press.

Richardson, A. (2001). *British romanticism and the science of the mind*. New York, NY: Cambridge University Press.

Rousseau, J. J. (1991). *Emile or on education*. London, England: Penguin Books.

Sharf, R. (2015). Is mindfulness Buddhist? (And why it matters). *Transcultural Psychiatry 52*(4), 470-484.

Springgay, S. (2008). *Body knowledge and curriculum: Pedagogies of touch in youth and visual culture*. New York, NY: Peter Lang.

Tabulawa, R. (2013). *Teaching and learning in context: Why pedagogical reforms fail in sub-Saharan Africa*. Dakar: CODESRIA.

Tavares, H. (2016). *Pedagogies of the image: Photo-archives, cultural histories, and post-foundational inquiry*. Dordrecht, the Netherlands: Springer.

Wokler, R. (1995). *Rousseau*. Oxford, England: Oxford University Press.

CHAPTER 2

SYNCOPATION, SENSING, AND SENSE-MAKING

The Genealogies of Julia Kristeva and Michel Foucault

David Lee Carlson
Mary Lou Fulton Teachers College

Joseph David Sweet
University of North Carolina at Pembroke

> Arizona State UniversityTo worry or to smile, such is the choice when we are assailed by the strange; our decision depends on how familiar we are with our own ghosts. (Kristeva, 1991, p. 191)

> Where religions once demanded the sacrifice of bodies, knowledge now calls for experimentation on ourselves, calls us to the sacrifice of the subject of knowledge. (Foucault, 1977, p. 163)

Scholars in the area of the sensuous curriculum present a rather strong case for the importance of the body in teaching and learning processes. Their work shifts the conversation in the field of curriculum studies from

Sensuous Curriculum:
Politics and the Senses in Education, pp. 29–45

cognitive discussions to more haptic understandings. Rather than produce scholarship absent affect, or sanitized from the body, sensory-oriented curriculum compels scholars to explore the epistemological and ontological modes that exceed the all too common cognitive function as the site of knowledge and experience. Scholars write about the intricacies of mothering, for example, and propose that "Sense-based theorizing asks less about what one thinks so much as it asks who one is, by the way of what one experiences, in their body as it moves through the world" (McDermott, 2011, p. 135). Other scholars writing in this area echo McDermott's emphasis on the body. They have written about how the role of art in classrooms generates "bodyful listening" (Weibe, 2011), how the history of museums historically guarded against touching physical objects, but holding and feeling an artifact actually helps museum-goers make sense of the world as well as feel and inspect their historical understandings (Wood & Latham, 2011), for example. Scholars have also discussed the role of disciplining procedures in schools and the sensory implications of those procedures (Leafgren, 2012), the relationship among food, identity, and sense-making (Hurren & Hasabe-Lubt, 2011). Additionally, scholars have focused on sound (Gershon, 2011), taste (Hurren & Hasabe-Lubt, 2011), touch (Wood & Latham, 2011), and somatic imagination (Fettes, 2011).

This chapter contributes to this burgeoning research and wishes to add to the line of work that explores the role history plays in the sensorium (Wood & Latham, 2011). Specifically, we propose a notion of ecstatic thinking under the umbrella of sensuous curriculum within the field of curriculum studies, an understanding grounded in James Bernauer's (1990) work on Foucault's ethical turn. Bernauer proposes that ecstatic thinking fosters an escape from oneself as a constructive personal affective project. We want to add to this literature by illustrating the relationship among genealogical history, the sensual, and ecstatic thinking. It is our argument that the sensorium, sensuality, and sense-making exceed the sociocultural framework. In fact, genealogical histories precede and thus demarcate the contours of the sociocultural map. More important, genealogical histories, or at least the ones discussed in this chapter, foster an escape from oneself as well as illustrate that senses and the sensuous can be more than the five senses. Genealogical senses and sense-making injects a discontinuous history into the discussion of how the senses work with and through the body.

What is at stake in this chapter is how curriculum scholars investigate the sensuous, the affective, and sense-making within the historical register. We seek to expand the limits of perspective beyond the sociocultural to include the historical. To these ends, problematizing the sociocultural and including a historical (genealogical) aspect to the sensorium is to expand the critical analytic tools scholars own to examine and explore role that sense-making and sensuality plays in the self-fashioning of the subject.

More concretely, we explore the genealogical analytics of Julia Kristeva and Michel Foucault to show how ecstatic thinking can be sensual experiences and as modes of sense-making. The syncopation of their historical analysis produces, or invites, ecstatic thinking as a sensory experience. Our use of the word "thought" refers to Nietzsche's argument that "thoughts are signs of a play and struggle of affects. They are always connected to their hidden roots" (2003, 1[75]). Thoughts as affect, as sensuality, move and are moving and have been moving from their discontinuous (historical) roots. Rather than representing an end point, historical roots illustrate a multidimensionality and transhistorical "play and struggle" of affects, of feelings, of senses, and of sense-making. Rather than relying on the Cartesian split, Nietzsche privileges the senses, in which affect functions as the catalysts for movements of thought. The "roots," or history that marks the body contained within each affective thought as a play of historical forces and of struggle, or a working out and a series of working tensions that emerge viscerally in the moment as assemblages of becomings (Nietzsche, 2003).

The purpose of this chapter is to explore the historical affects of sensusous curriculum. The sensorium in many respects is a collection of thought embodied in a series of play and struggle that materialized in the affective dimensions. Thus, we pose the following question: What part does history play in a sensuous curriculum? To answer this question this chapter explicates Julia Kristeva's (1991) *Strangers to Ourselves* and Michel Foucault's (1977) genealogical analytic in "Nietzsche, Genealogy, and History" as a critique of Enlightenment and to propose the possibility of ecstatic thought within a sensory curriculum. Kristeva and Foucault's genealogical proposals offer scholars in the field of curriculum studies doing research on sensuous curriculum ways to explore how historical practices and rationalities implant themselves on the body, in the affect of sensuous curriculum.

Genealogy fosters ecstatic thinking because it invites readers to delay or place in abeyance their preconceived, taken-for-granted notions and practices in the present moment and about the present moment, a point of understanding shared in both Kristeva and Foucault's approaches. Furthermore, both of their approaches illustrate ways in which history operates on and through the body (sensual) in the present moment. Furthermore, both Kristeva and Foucault launch serious critiques of the Enlightenment and of humanism, arguments that appear to counter the preference for socio-culture theory privileged by scholars of sensuous curriculum (see below). Rather than show a progressive history, Kristeva (1991) offers a genealogical historical *toccata/fugue* to argue for Europeans to reconcile the "uncanny strangeness" (p. 187) within themselves in relation to others in order to quell violent tendencies towards foreigners as well as to live cosmopolitan lives. Complimenting such understandings, Foucault's genealogical analytic continually problematizes discourses and practices as play and struggle in the affective of the taken-for-granted of the present moment, a constant provocation of the sensual and sense-making that involves continually contesting notions of progress, the pseudo-sciences, and the mechanistic aspects of power/knowledge.

The chapter unfolds in the following manner. First, we unpack some of the main tenants of the sensual curriculum using Gershon's (2011) landmark article in *Journal of Curriculum Theorizing*, the article that provides the theoretical foundation for the field of the sensual curriculum prior to this volume, including Gershon's updating of those possibilities and pathways. Next, we present Kristeva's (1991) book *Strangers to Ourselves*, paying particular attention to its genealogical approach of strangeness/foreignness. Central to this approach is an illustration of how Kristeva uses history to produce a sensual curriculum that privileges the corporeal over the cognitive, genealogical strangeness that gets worn on the body in the "strange uncanny" (p. 192). Next, the chapter attends to Michel Foucault's (1977) genealogical analytic with particular attention to his essay, "Nietzsche, Genealogy, and History" because it is generally understood to be the philosophical foundation of Foucault's genealogical analytic (Dreyfus & Rabinow, 1983; Prado, 1995; Koopman, 2013). This section is followed by a discussion of the ways in which Foucault's genealogical history produces ecstatic thinking and, in so doing, also produces the visceral over the cognitive. We conclude the chapter with comments about the historical aspects of the sensorium and potential directions for the field of curriculum studies.

SENSUOUS CURRICULUM

Scholars who conduct research in the area of the sensual curriculum seek to examine the course of processes that individuals and groups enact to live sensual lives. As such, they continually make sense of phenomenon and of ineffable bodily experiences that are perceived through their senses. Sense-making and sensing the world are both individual experiences and socioculturally constructed. One's individual repertoire of both making sense of things and sensing the body in the world is determined partially by the social environment or local situatedness as well as one's cultural place. In this way, how one makes sense of one's senses becomes a political act. It can either disrupt or reinforce oppressive and repressive forms of power.

As a curriculum, sensuality privileges bodily senses, so sense-making of perceptions and experiences are personal predilections, which are favored over more cognitive ways of making sense. Thought remains fluid, and multifaceted rather than concrete, stable, and static. Knowledge, then, is co-constructed by several competing and complimentary factors. Gershon (2011) points out that while the sensual curriculum focuses on the senses, it "does not preclude critical attention to texts or its use in order to represent ideas, concepts, and constructs" (p. 2). In fact, including senses in the sense-making process expands the potential ways of knowing, and sensual curriculum ties ontology to epistemology through the body. The course of one's learning links affect with thought and feelings with cognition and senses with making sense. Hence, it injects the sense with affect into the meaning-making endeavor, and affect precedes cognition in the course of the teaching and learning process.

The sensual curriculum contains neither solely the aesthetic nor just the political but generates a "nexus of meaning making and the sense in curriculum studies" (Gershon, 2011, p. 2). It is an "open, fluid framework of possibilities" (Gershon, 2011, p. 2). It can combine the aesthetic with the political in that it offers experiences and perceptions through and with the body that carry the potential to contest privileged and normalized ways of knowing. The sensual curriculum can provide students with opportunities to make sense of the world through their senses that contest the reproduction of dominant discourses and hierarchies. Possibilities drive and in some cases replace reproduction of power arrangements. In this way, the sensual curriculum is always-already in process, or in-the-making. It is an emergent relational and at times ineffable process that defies representations and the claws of formal knowledge. It is an embodied experience of making sense. Not knowledge as decomposed (Ellsworth, 1997).

The nexus between embodied curriculum and knowledge production is grounded primarily in French philosophical thoughts. Due to the turn recently to the sensual, French thinkers "pursue the ways in which the sensual is political in thought and action" (Gershon, 2011, p. 7). To summarize, the sensuous curriculum embodies a sociocultural perspective and a constructivist epistemology. What constitutes senses and sense making are constructed with various emergent factors. This means that there are no transcendental or essentialized historical senses or methods of sense-making, so there are no hierarchies of senses or ways of knowing. Finally, the epistemological and methodological perspectives and constructs inform the modalities of representation and scholarship in the field of curriculum studies. Sensuous curriculum can function as political acts that extend and contest taken-for-granted ways of knowing and being in the world.

The very notion of "text" in the sensuous curriculum becomes reconceptualized. Rather than distinguishing between senses and textuality, scholars in the burgeoning field of sensuous curriculum contend that the senses are texts and contain their own thought, produce their own ideas, concepts and constructs. As texts, they emerge with historical traces genealogically rather than constructed socioculturally. The historical ontology of the genealogical analytic reveals itself in the processes of sense-making through the senses. History seeps through the body and through the senses and/or simultaneously with thought. Rather than disciplining or constructing the sense-making of the senses, a genealogical approach contends that the sensual curriculum emerges through a variation and sometimes unknowable assemblages of historical contingencies that challenge sense-making in the present moment. The genealogical approach inserts the notion of archival chance in the potentialities of the sensuous curriculum and the sensorium becomes problematized in its historical variability and (dis)continuities. Rather than construct history as a grand narrative, genealogical studies focus on the ruptures of history in order to challenge taken-for-granted notions and practices of the present moment. Genealogies are not total histories; they are specific histories of specific practices designed to excavate the gaps and fissures neglected in grand narratives in order to reveal the machinations of power/knowledge on the body.

The purpose, or what's at stake in our analysis, is what we call the ecstatic curriculum, a course that fosters an escape of oneself as a fashioning of the self. Rather than a sociocultural construct, the ecstatic sensuous curriculum emerges, flows, moves, acts, and thinks in historical variability in the present moment. The ecstatic sensuous curriculum injects an archival exploration into the modes of knowledge production that allows individuals to contest and subvert dominate forms of knowledge. The ecstatic sensuous curriculum fosters a distance from oneself in order to produce self-disorientation moving fluidly in the process of self-invention or being an ecstatic self-in-the-making. It also extends the sensuous beyond the five senses to the potentiality of genealogical senses and sense-making, where multiple ineffable, ill-defined sense and sense-making occurs ongoing and in-the-making.

FUGUE, TOCCATA, AND GENEALOGY

Our move towards what ecstatic sensuous curriculum might mean and how it can function begins with Julia Kristeva's *Strangers to Ourselves* (1991). Kristeva explores the history of the foreigner and his/her strangeness in four different historical periods, one that neither produces a grand or total narrative about foreigners, nor seeks to produce a unified theory of "the foreigner." Instead, she offers a reading of the foreigner in order to displace the reader's perspective about their own reluctances to their own strangeness/foreignness. Embracing strangeness, its history and bodily experiences, Kristeva contends, illustrates how foreigners make sense, or, conversely, allows one to embrace one's own strangeness. As she does with history, Kristeva does not level out or produce a hierarchy of strangeness but recognizes how one appears as strange or other in the world of differences. Recognizing difference, strangeness, and the foreigner within invites escape, or the allure to interact with the strange and foreign within oneself as well as in the world. Combining the psychological known of strangeness with cultural foreignness illustrates how psychoanalysis contains a political function. Moreover, it is often through the understanding of one's psychological strangeness as an unknown that one is invited to explore the foreigner.

The history of the escape explicated in her book and the potential for ecstatic thinking comes with both costs and rewards—sometimes simultaneously. Through her genealogical investigation of the foreigner, Kristeva invites the reader to explore the potential for escaping oneself. Kristeva's style, on the other hand, reflects what she calls a *Toccata*, which is commonly associated with musical performances to represent a free-style approach to show off the musician's touch. For example, where her book reflects the *Toccata* style in that the first half section collects a series of historical examples of foreigners as descriptors of how foreignness has been conceived and understood thematically, the second half functions much closer to her definition of fugue. The fugue, according to Kristeva, in psychiatric terms represents a loss of identity and a flight from one's normal, everyday environment. To experience or recognize strangeness in oneself through and with others is a perfect illustration of a *Fugue*. The free-style of the Toccata with the affect of the Fugue illustrates the ecstatic potentialities of Kristeva's genealogy of the stranger. More important, they (Toccata and Fugue) provide the reader with an opportunity to experience moments of self-escape; to reconsider strangeness and its affects. The genealogy of toccata and fugue offers the reader to generate their own ecstatic sensual curriculum.

To read Kristeva's work is to confront and identify with the strange sensuality of being a foreigner, as well as to reconsider the strangeness of sense-making. The curriculum or course, in the book resembles a *Fugue*, in its polyphonic arrangement of various themes from multiple perspectives containing contrapuntal components leading or merging several somewhat distinct divisions to a definitive climax at its conclusion. The *fugue* as a concept is also used in psychiatry to describe a person who experiences a period of memory loss and yet begins life anew through the amnesic escape. The feeling of escape through the amnesic moment permits the person to emerge strange to oneself and thus to begin life anew. The *fugue* fragments time. It (Fugue) is incomplete, discontinuous (amnesia) and belies linear historical trajectories. It seeks experience by recalling memories about the foreigner, and builds a new life grounded in one's strangeness. Kristeva's curriculum or course of history as outlined in her book serves as a *Fugue* for the reader. Her genealogy of the foreigner puts the reader in a momentary slumber, making them forget who they think they are in order to inspire a renewed relationships to the foreigner and thus one's own strangeness. As Kristeva (1991) states in the following quote,

> Let us not seek to solidify, to turn the otherness of the foreigner into a thing. Let us merely touch it, brush by it, without giving it a permanent structure. Simply sketching out is perpetual motion through some of its variegated aspects spread out before our eyes today, through some of its former, changing representations scattered throughout history. Let us also lighten the otherness by constantly coming back to it—but more and more swiftly. Let us escape its hatred, its burden, fleeing them not through leveling and forgetting, but through the harmonious repletion of the differences it implies and spreads. Toccatas and Fugues: Bach's compositions evoke to my ears the meaning of an acknowledged and harrowing otherness that I should like to be contemporary, because it has been brought up, relieved, disseminated, inscribed in an original play being developed, without goal, without boundary, without end. An otherness barely touched up and that barely moves away. (p. 3)

Forgetting is a sensual, bodily experience as well as a form of sense-making as it is in remembering to touch and to "sketching out its perpetual motion through some of its variegated aspects" (p. 3). This sketching fosters a new sense-making, to *not* dehumanize the other, the foreigner, or "turn ... the foreigner into a thing" (p. 3). She offers the reader the opportunity to defer their current. entrenched understandings of the foreigner in order to "touch it, brush by it" (p. 3) and to traverse the "harmonious depletion" (p. 3) of its (foreigner) various historical narratives. Kristeva implores her readers to explore the historical narratives of the foreigner, not through "leveling and forgetting," but through an immersion in the differences that persist between the "foreigner" and the "native." Kristeva's reminder of the divergent historical themes and narratives about the foreigner readers to confront their own strangeness and to modify how they view the foreigner in the present moment. What do the harmonious repetitions teach us? What are the sensuous experiences, or the sensorium of the foreigner according to Kristeva? How does her genealogical project of the foreigner aid the reader to develop an ecstatic curriculum? The next section of the paper answers these questions.

In the first section of her book, Kristeva (1991) tackles the problem of the relationship between the foreigner and native within the context of European nationalism. The foreigner, she exclaims, challenges the common sense and entrenched perspective that buttresses and privileges the European nationalistic identity. The European's willingness to accept internal strangeness within themselves in order to understand the plight of the foreigner becomes crucial to adapting to the new European landscape:

"By recognizing him (foreigner) within ourselves, we are spared detesting him [foreigner]in himself" (p. 1). This construct of the foreigner can be understood as pertaining to one of two overarching themes, the foreigner in relation to his/her body and the foreigner in relation to place, understandings to which we now turn our focus.

To those who perceive themselves to be entitled to a strong sense of European nationalism, the foreigner's body represents an intrusion, a moment of profound, explicit interrupting difference with the potential for exile. The foreigner's face represents an intrusive trace that affronts the ordinary citizen. This affront disrupts a (false) sense of normalcy, a generally known sense of the enclosed, hermetic European world, as well as representing risky possibilities for alternative modes of being in the world—the foreigner's face invites the possibilities for community based on difference that is both frightening and thrilling. To further this point, Kristeva (1991) states, "Living with the other, with the foreigner, confronts us with the possibility or not of *being an other*. It is not simply—humanistically—a matter of our being able to accept the other, but of *being in his place*, and this means to imagine and make oneself other for oneself" (p. 13). Where the foreigner exposes the otherness within European nationalists and activates the strangeness within them, the foreigner's body represents opportunities that provoke self-risk, self-displacement, and the urge to self-solidify in the face of differences, constructed and visible.

In terms of place, the foreigner represents the continual wanderer and the one who remains in exile, one who leaves, abandoning all ties to the motherland, and seeks the promise land. The foreigner's understanding of an origin remains faulty and inconsequential as "The strange happiness of the foreigner consists in maintaining that fleeing eternity or that perpetual transience" (Kristeva, 1991, p. 4). The foreigner maintains no grip or hold on certainty of an origin; they accept the inevitability of change. The foreigner symbolizes the evanescence of life to the native. The promise lands forever in his/her dreams and remains continually beyond his/her comprehension. Their origin lost, or hidden, the foreigner strives to take root in the new place but keeps the "present in abeyance" (Kristeva, 1991, p. 7), a combination that can make the foreigner seem aloof, detached, and nonplussed by the waving vagaries of the unfamiliar terrain.

Psychologically, the foreigner's strangeness emerges at the time of his mother's death, Kristeva (1991) surmises, when separation from the mother and the origin is lost and wandering begins, separated by from the motherland. As the foreigner commences the journey to the land of forever in the elsewhere, a sense of displacement ensues, and the place of the other emerges. It is then that we, natives and foreigners alike struggle to move about and through the world of difference. The foreigner and native mingle in a continual flow of difference. In contrast, Kristeva argues that, for the foreigner, natives "have not life at all: barely do they exist, haughty or mediocre, but out of the running and thus almost already cadaverized" (p. 7). The bodies of natives who strive to sanitize difference through their work to eradicate the presence of difference appear delusional, repressed, and dead to the foreigner; they (natives) enclose and obstruct the risky possibilities of community and communion with others. More important they fail to recognize the potential for living and remaining in exile, for "The strangeness of the European begins with his inner exile" (p. 26). The fractured and fissured body of the exile unleashes itself from the repressive regimes that provoke the exile to seek a new land. That repression of the former land can become transferred to the new place, and even though the foreigner thinks he has "outsmarted" it remains "moving around perfidiously, on a lower level, on the borders between soma and psyche, where the sluice gates of *jouissance* become snagged and unleashed eroticism is obliged to resort to new limits, those of organs, which then falters" (p. 31). The dreams of the new horizon confront the limits of the strange place as the libidinal rules shift and remain constricted in a yet much different fashion. The exotic wanderings of the foreigner function as a fold for the native of both their (native) own strangeness and the desire for the other. The foreigner serves as the catalyst for libidinal possibilities. The distinction between the native and the foreigner remain a bit heavy-handed, only to be mitigate by Kristeva's ironic tone. She places the foreigner and the native in a binary position only to illustrate their inter-relatedness. The foreigner and the native merge in the possibilities of the strange uncanny. In this instance, then, the foreigner and the native coexist in a continual world of difference; one that fosters a youthful cosmopolitanism bolstered by discontinuity and a fractured identity.

It is the openness to the shifting of libininal rules and the potential for fresh insights and novel experiences that produce the possibilities for a youthful cosmopolitanism, the characteristics of one who "shelters a shattered origin" (Kristeva, 1991, p. 38) and revels in the nomadic life beyond the nation-state. The cosmopolitan figure defies stability and reviews the past with a dubious and cleft eye. In short, the cosmopolitan individual exists in a continual state of *Tocatta/Fugue,* a discontinuous syncopation of amnesia and renewal. The youthful cosmopolitan person releases the understanding they have of themselves in order to fashion a different one. So much so that they "succeed in viewing ourselves as unessential, simple passerby, retaining of the past only the game" (Kristeva, 1991, p. 38). Kristeva's provocation about European cosmopolitanism portrayed by a sense of touching the "untouchable void" instigates the questions, what accounts for this cosmopolitanism? What does the strangeness within ourselves afford us within this cosmopolitanism?

COSMOPOLITANISM AND FOREIGNNESS

To answer these questions, Kristeva (1991) completes an incomplete and discontinuous genealogy of foreigners throughout various historical periods. Due to the limitations of the chapter, we have elected to focus our attention on the Enlightenment and Kristeva's turn toward the strange "uncanny" within us. To do so, Kristeva moves from the historical to the psychological register in order to arouse a sense-making prompted by ecstatic thinking, or, in her terms, as a continual escaping of the self exemplified in relations between native and foreigner. The genealogical project as an incomplete history and as an inescapable tacking back and forth between fugue and toccata kindles a wandering *of* the self *on* and *by* the self. Although Kristeva's approach to genealogy differs in subtle and important ways from Foucault's, their application of the genealogy remains quite similar. For Kristeva, genealogy begins with a critique of the relationship between cosmopolitanism and the foreigner in the present moment.

Kristeva (1991) argues that a modern conception of natural and political man emerges during the Enlightenment. Kristeva argues that a fundamental "splitting" between the citizen and the noncitizen, a differentiation that, in turn, establishes the conditions between native and foreigner. It is this declaration that provokes Kirsteva to wonder if cosmopolitanism can function or exists with the foreigner and, more importantly, troubles our understanding of nationalism in the present moment. In response, citing Arendt, Kristeva argues that Enlightenment ideals collapses during the Nazi regime, where the status of man proved insufficient to ensure citizenship and all of its supposed promises. Turning to psychoanalysis as a means to challenge the spirit of the Enlightenment in the abstract and its promises of the universal man (Beardsworth, 2004), Kristeva contends that the spirit must be replaced with the ways in which humanity actually works.

> One would notice, in addition to the social propensity for association and life, murderous surges, *jouissance* of death, pleasures of parting and narcissism, carrier waves of the social fabric's fragmentation but also that of the very identity of the individuals' body and their psychic space. The destructive tendencies of society come together with those that destroy human nature as well as human biology and the individual's identity. (pp. 152–153)

It is the reality of how humans actually behave, rather than assumptions about how they could do so, that causes Kristeva to simultaneously argue against the abstract principles in the *Enlightenment* and for the unrelated tools of psychoanalysis linked to an ethics of "strange uncanny" (p. 178). It is education that Kristeva believes to be an appropriate pathway to explore the strangeness of man while building a sense of cosmopolitanism that invites the foreign/strange both within and among us. In short, Kristeva argues for the emergence of a culture that fosters difference and foreignness as opposed to the rather German ideal of collapsing the self-formation of the *bildung* to promote a nationalists (closed) identity. To these ends, she endorses an education that fosters a multilayered, complex understanding of oneself and the world through and with an other, Freud's discussion of "uncanny strangeness," or on our estimation an ecstatic curriculum that fosters self-escape instigated by genealogical analysis.

The "strange uncanny" incites "many variations" and "repeat(s) the difficulty I have in situating myself with respect to the other and keep going over the course of identification-projection that lies at the foundation of my reading autonomy" (Kristeva, 1991, p. 187). Kristeva (1991) reminds us that Freud does not discuss strangeness per se, but invites us to "detect foreignness in ourselves" (p. 191) so that we may not "hound it outside us" (p. 191). It is the uncanny strangeness that invites a cosmopolitanism that blurs boundaries and one grounded in the understanding that one's unconscious urges and desires drive consciousness. It is a cosmopolitanism that is built on a bewildering difference that necessitates an acceptance of the otherness of ourselves. It is an understanding of what is a "strange uncanny" that can be used to actively invite a sense of strangeness within ourselves *so that* we may be with others in harmonious ways. A genealogical project is designed to disorient and to instigate an ecstatic sensuous experience.

Conversely, genealogical *Fugue* established by Kristeva (1991) illustrates how recognizing the strangeness within ourselves permits us to invite the foreigner. It is the continual engagement with the uncanny that one explores the experiments with the possibilities of one's humanity. The genealogy exhibit by Kristeva reflects the strangeness described in her book: both the form and content match. The purpose of the genealogy is to provoke dissonance in reader's understanding of the stranger in order to ignite the reader's "strange uncanny." In this way, then, the genealogy operates on the body through the excitation of the uncanny through the body. It is the understanding of various historical approaches to the foreigner/stranger that one realizes that differences instigates the necessary conditions for community.

Foucault's Genealogy as Fictional Sketch

Michel Foucault (1977) uses history to problematize the production of truth based on common knowledge practices in the present moment. Like Kristeva, he neither composes a grand narrative nor produces a theory of power. Instead, he exposes the historical contingencies and machinations of power on the body, responding to a rather different foe in his genealogical analysis. Instead of contesting European nationalism, in *Nietzsche, Genealogy, History* (1977), Foucault argues that historians such as Paul Ree reduce the history of morality to a quest for unity through a linear movement towards a unified historical narrative. According to Foucault, Ree

> assumed that words had kept their meaning, that desires still pointed in a single direction, and that ideas retained their logic; and he ignored the fact that the world of speech and desires has known invasions, struggles, plundering, disguises, ploys. (p. 139)

Instead, history and meaning through language involve a complex system of moves that resemble a continual and chaotic war more than a linear and sequential and relatively even progression. For these reasons, Foucault maintains that genealogy must seek events that exist in the affective, in "unpromising places" such as "in sentiments, love, conscience, instincts; it must be sensitive to their recurrence, not in order to trace the gradual curve of their evolution, but to isolate the different scenes where they engage in different roles" (pp. 139–140). Genealogies, thus, do not seek origins, but persist in their singularities.

Chance rather than continuity and streamlining historical events become more important to pursue in the genealogical analysis. For the genealogist, there are no ahistorical, essentialized unrevealed unities. What is found at the origin is disparity. Progressive historians, Foucault (1977) asserts, assume that the origin precedes the body, the world and time. On the contrary, Foucault claims, origins are "lowly" "derisive and ironic, capable of undoing every infatuation" (p. 143). The origin precedes all knowledge or represents a return to the original, pure form of knowledge and truth, but from Foucault's perspective, the origin reflects a sense of loss due to its overabundance of possibilities and "excesses of its own speech" (p. 143). In Kristevian terms, the genealogists is a foreigner, and from Foucault's perspective, purposefully places herself in the position of disorientation in order to ignite the senses. The process of doing a genealogy, then, itself is an ecstatic experience, a self-disorienting process.

The genealogy searches for the minute details and the accidents that permit certain regimes of truth to emerge. Rather than coalescing major historical events, such as wars, great leaders, and major demographical shifts, the genealogists unearths the "petty malice(s)" (Foucault, 1977, p. 144) of history that reveals the emergence of certain practices and discourses of power/knowledge on the body. The genealogist focuses on the body, "its conditions, of weakness and strength, its breakdown and resistances, to be in a position to judge philosophical discourse" (Foucault, 1977, p. 145). Thus, instead of searching for the one origin, the genealogist seeks the numberless beginnings as a sifting out of disparities that occur during any epoch.

Building from Nietzsche's work in the *Genealogy of Morals* (1968), Foucault (1977) discusses two themes of Nietzsche's important treatise. The first, the descent, or *Herkunft*, produces a "dissociation of the self" and its understanding of one's past as well as one's identity. Identity is not a unifying characteristic for Foucault, but is an amalgamation of various entities, many unknown, but shifting and porous and in constant motion. Historical practices and discourses as discontinuity produce a self in its disparity and soaked in chance and accidents. One's heritage does not grow and calcify, but is an "unstable assemblage of faults, fissures, and heterogeneous layers that threaten the fragile inheritor from within or from underneath" (p. 146). Decent as an assemblage, then, attaches itself to the body, "It inscribes itself in the nervous system, in temperament, in the digestive apparatus; it appears in faulty respiration, in improper diets, in the debilitated and prostrate body of those whose ancestors committed errors" (p. 147).

Therefore, historically contingent factors infringe on the body and "gives rise to desires, failings, and errors" (Foucault, 1977, p. 148). The body becomes the "inscribed surface" of historical events as well as the "the locus of a dissociated self, and a volume in perpetual disintegration" (Foucault, 1977, p. 148). The body remains both a doing and an undoing of the self as it continually engages with historical contingencies that seek shape it in the present moment, or as a foreigner/native as strange uncanny in a Kristevian sense. Thus, the purpose of a genealogy is to chart the ways in which historical events embed themselves in the body as well as shows the "process of history's destruction of the body" (Foucault, 1977, p. 148). The genealogist shows how the human sciences (e.g., psychology; criminology; pedagogy) destroy the body as it simultaneously strives to construct it.

The second aspect to Foucault's (1977) analysis of Nietzsche's genealogy is emergence, or *Entstehung*. Emergence describes how historical events culminate not as a stopping point, but as "a series of subjugations" (p. 148). The genealogist illustrates or describes perilous and agonistic play of multiple forces of dominations. The purpose of the emergences is to describe this continual and constant play of various forces within a historical period as well as to trace its innumerable beginnings and its ebbs and flows throughout history. Genealogies in their singularities depict and map the tangled web of practices of power that infringe and demarcate the body in various historical situations. The subject may be the outcome, but the body remains the target of power/knowledge. Disciplinary practices, for example, of schooling hit the body and thus have sensuous effects. The play of dominations within power production and knowledge formation occurs in historical moments where some forms of domination strengthen and then weaken; certain rationalities along with specific practices appear in certain historical moments and then refashion themselves in others based on some known and unknown conditions. The point here is that emergence in the Foucauldian genealogical analytic describes, or diagnoses, these alterations in order to reveal the machinations of power/knowledge on truth and ultimately on the production of the subject through the body. The field of emergences remains open, fluid, flexible. Emergences shows the contestations of various discourses and practices on the body in order to produce a certain type of subject in a specific space; and to produce knowledge about the subject.

The genealogist seeks to understand and more deeply engage the taken-for-granted sayable and knowable about the subject as a history of the present. As an incomplete, but critical history, the genealogy operates on the assumption that historical narratives resemble a fictional sketch. The archival fragments assembled by the genealogists illustrate the play of dominations as power/knowledge in order to contest, subvert and historically deconstruct grand narratives or claims to metaphysical certainty. Progressive humanists' historical narratives collapse in the face of the petty, raucous, and cacophonous archival shimmy of the genealogist. The purpose of the genealogies is to illustrate that what is currently taken-for-granted is not necessarily the "best" or superior, or even the morally right way to do things, to be a human being. Foucault provokes readers to remain aware of the dangers of power/knowledge formations and offers readers opportunities at invention, experimentation, and curiosity. As Foucault (1977) exclaims,

> We believe, in any event, that the body obeys the exclusive laws of physiology and that it escapes the influence of history, but this too is false. The body is modeled by a great many distinct regimes; it is broke down by the rhythms of work, rest and holidays; it is poisoned by food or values, through eating habits or moral laws; it constructs resistances. (p. 153)

The body does not escape history but is in fact informed and partially shaped by a variety of historically contingent forces.

Michel Foucault's (1977) genealogical project seeks to show how discontinuous and fragmented historical narratives shape and demarcate the subject through the body. Machinations of power/knowledge agonistically wrestle with each other to try to direct the body in certain ways, but the battle never ends. It is through conducting a genealogy and reading his works that the reader learns about the movements of power/knowledge of the subject and truth through the body that the reader can learn and understand how to adjust and adapt to specific forms of power/knowledge. The genealogy remains an incomplete history trespassing normalized demarcations of formal knowledge in a contentious field that strives to guide the affectual aspects and experiences of the body. Knowledge operates in and through the body in its historical contingencies and shiftiness. The syncopation of the genealogy provides for moments of self-escape, or ecstatic thinking. Ecstatic thinking occurs through the genealogical process in the understanding of the ways and means of the effects of power/knowledge on the body.

CONCLUSION

The syncopation of both Kristeva and Foucault's genealogies illustrate the ways in which history implants itself in the affective domains to produce sense-making through the senses and the body. Kristeva's (1991) urge to engage with the always-already uncanny within oneself invites the reader to continually engage with the strange and with the foreigner in order to generate a sense of community. Foucault's (1977) genealogical analytic illustrates the machinations of power/knowledge and how they persist on and through the body as a continual war among various historical forces of domination. He argues that disparity and discontinuity belie claims for metaphysical certainty and historical unity. The subject is a production of power/knowledge and it is through the affective that this production occurs.

The ecstatic thinking that occurs throughout both genealogies illustrates how historical investigations can produce a disorientation of the body. Ecstatic thinking as a play and struggle through the affect occurs when one repositions oneself and thus disorientates oneself in order to sense relationships in a new way. This type of engagement then offers alternative possibilities for sense-making, and thus altering the sensorium. The genealogy as a form is foreign; it defies methodology, and puts the archivists in a strange position of uncertainty and risk. The genealogist perseveres in the unknown and confronts the uncanny, or strangeness within him/herself. By conducting a genealogy, the researchers engage in ecstatic thinking because it forces them to leave one, or to confront one's strangeness. The genealogical endeavor remains a visceral, vibrational, and chaotic bodily experience as taken-for-granted notions become troubled. The once known solidified self begins to fissure, crack, and fragment. Kristeva (1991) admonishes the reader to face the strangeness within oneself and to live in the uncomfortable position of corporal dissonance. Foucault (1977), on the other hand, urges readers to dive into the discontinuity and live the alterity. The necessity to explore the critical history and to embody the genealogical analytic to expose the strategies of power/knowledge remains vital for Foucault. He insists that we must remain strange to ourselves and embrace uncertainty in the face of the always-already whims of chance. The affective aspects of the sensual curriculum necessitate a greater exploration into the sociocultural aspects and the historical ones, too.

REFERENCES

Beardsworth, S. (2004). *Julia Kristeva: Psychoanalysis and modernity*. Albany, NY: State University of New York Press.

Bernauer, J. W. (1990). *Michel Foucault's force of flight: Toward an ethics for thought*. Amherst, NY: Humanity Books.

Dreyfus, H. L., & Rabinow, P. (1983). *Michel Foucault: Beyond structuralism and hermeneutics* (2nd ed.). Chicago, IL: The University of Chicago Press.

Ellsworth, E. (1997). *Teaching positions: Difference, pedagogy, and the power of address*. New York, NY: Teachers College Press.

Foucault, M. (1977). Nietzsche, genealogy, history. In D. F. Bouchard (Ed.), *Language, counter-memory, practices: Selected essays and interviews by Michel Foucault* (pp. 139–164). Ithaca, NY: Cornell University Press.

Fettes, M. (2011). Senses and sensibilities: Educating the somatic imagination. *JCT (Online)*, *27*(2), 114.

Gershon, W. S. (2011). Embodied knowledge: Sounds as educational systems. *JCT (Online)*, *27*(2), 66–81.

Hurren, W., & Hasebe-Ludt, E. (2011). Bringing curriculum down to earth: The terror that we are. *JCT (Online)*, *27*(2), 17–34.

Koopman, C. (2013). *Genealogy as critique: Foucault and the problems of modernity*. Bloomington and Indianapolis, IN: Indiana University Press.

Kristeva, J. (1991). *Strangers to ourselves*. New York, NY: Columbia University Press.

Leafgren, S. L. (2011). " Hands at your sides!" The severing of body and mind in the elementary school. *JCT (Online)*, *27*(2), 35–50.

McDermott, M. (2011). Curriculum of the eye/I. *JCT (Online)*, *27*(2), 130–144.

Nietzsche, F. (1968). *Genealogy of morals*. In W. Kaufmann (Ed.), *Basic writings of Nietzsche* (pp. 451–599). New York, NY: The Modern Library.

Nietzsche, F. (2003). *Nietzsche: Writings from the late notebooks*. Cambridge, MA: Cambridge University Press.

Prado, C.G. (1995). *Starting with Foucault: An introduction to genealogy*. Boulder, CO: Westview Press.

Wiebe, S., & Snowber, C. (2011). The visceral imagination: A fertile space for non-textual knowing. *JCT (Online)*, *27*(2), 101–113.

Wood, E., & Latham, K. F. (2011). The thickness of things: Exploring the curriculum of museums through phenomenological touch. *JCT (Online)*, *27*(2), 51–65.

CHAPTER 3

WELCOMING WHAT WE CANNOT IMAGINE

Sensory Curriculum in Teacher Education

Lee Airton
Faculty of Education, Queen's University

In this chapter, I discuss some pedagogical implications for teacher education stemming from my recent dissertation (Airton, 2014) on social justice teacher education or SJTE. I define the work of SJTE as preparing teachers to welcome and foster social difference, but it is more commonly defined as preparing teachers to practice in a way that narrows demographic divides in education, including that between privileged students on the one hand and historically underserved students on the other (see Airton, 2014). The academic field of SJTE is largely American despite having considerable influence in Canada and around the world. It is a deeply historical and venerable field, with a recognizable pantheon (e.g., James Banks, Geneva Gay, Carl Grant, Sonia Nieto, Christine Sleeter, Anna-Maria Villegas) and canon (e.g., Grant & Secada's 1990 foundational literature review on preparing teachers for diversity, or Villegas and Lucas' 2002 book on preparing culturally relevant teachers). Crucially, SJTE is beset by perpetual anxiety about its difference from other approaches to teacher

Sensuous Curriculum:
Politics and the Senses in Education, pp. 47–66

education. In other words, if teacher educators who prepare future teachers for "social justice practice" have been successful—if we have produced "social justice teachers"—how do we know? How will the outcome of this work differ from the outcome of teacher education approaches that do *not* do the things prioritized in the SJTE literature?

Seasoned SJTE field leaders and more recent commentators alike have asked these questions for over 20 years (e.g., Cochran-Smith, Davis, & Fries, 2004; Dover, 2009; Gorski, 2010; Grant & Secada, 1990; Hollins & Guzman, 2005; Ladson-Billings, 1995; Zeichner, 2009) and found the literature wanting in empirical answers. Because and/or in spite of this absence, the SJTE literature bristles with yardsticks: principles, definitions and attributes of "real SJTE." Intended to be stable across diverse teacher education contexts, these yardsticks are held to gauge whether a program "truly" prepares students for the work of social justice teaching. Here, language is often used as a proxy for the "real SJTE" that cannot be empirically measured; proxies can include: (a) whether programs or practitioners use terms like privilege, oppression and systemic *inter alia* racism, or "settle for lesser terms" like tolerance and equality; (b) whether (and where, or how close to the beginning) particular topics are listed on course syllabi; (c) whether a standalone "social justice" course is listed in the calendar or, better still, required; or (d) what words appear (and where, or how close to the beginning) in program mission statements (see Ahmed, 2012; Airton, 2014). But can these language-based proxies signal that a teacher education approach is *actually, materially* about "social justice," or, that it *is* social justice teacher education and not just teacher education in social justice clothing? Moreover, can the difference between these two things ever be known?

In constructing my research problem, I argued that SJTE's identity headache is in fact methodological. It is nigh-on impossible to show that SJTE is empirically different from "non-social-justice" approaches to teacher education because the requisite evidence is impossible to produce within dominant positivism-inspired frameworks. "Social justice" simply will not behave like a stable outcome: an end from which we can look backwards and confer retroactive value on a process now found worthy of further time and resource investment, most often through some form of measurement. Even if "social justice" did somehow arrive, this would spell the obsolescence of SJTE because it would cease to be needed.

Nevertheless, the everyday work of SJTE—or "teaching the diversity class," as this work is commonly and wryly characterized—carries on in the service of "social justice,"' something paradoxically conceived as *far* from the teacher education classroom in space and time yet *near enough* that it can be affected by what we will have done together, today. In the face of this problem, it is rather wondrous that a field with such a defining yet impossible outcome as "social justice" is able to stay together and keep working when it cannot pin down the outcomes of its difficult labor. Some might say that SJTE is at risk of failure because it cannot definitively demonstrate its outcome, a message as likely to be found within SJTE as without (e.g., Cochran-Smith, Barnatt, Lahann, Shakman, & Terrell, 2009).

Instead of joining the quest for empirical evidence to support SJTE's difference-as-existence, I decentered dominant quantitative logics that privilege measurability, replicability and generalizability at the expense of the local, emergent, and singular. I also decentered dominant qualitative frameworks that tend to erase the gap between language (whether in a text or a transcript) and event as though these are one and the same: for example, that what an interviewee says about their experience in a formal interview equals their experience (see Mazzei, 2004, 2009). Instead of relying on what SJTE scholars say or write about the field and its task, I turned to neo-materialism and post-qualitative methodology (see Lather, 2013; Lather & St. Pierre, 2013; St. Pierre, 2013) to otherwise explore what might actually, materially keep SJTE together as an identifiable field. As I hope to show in the following pages, this turn enabled me to argue that the field of SJTE is an *assemblage* (Deleuze & Guattari, 1987, 1996)—a provisional whole without a static identity across time and space—and that, therefore, the practice of SJTE is an *affective craft*. It is an undertaking that requires the modulation of affect, in the Massumian (2002) sense of sensation or intensity. I concluded my dissertation with some suggestions on how to do this modulation, or, how to use rises and falls in affective intensity in the teacher education classroom. his chapter represents a personal next step in the evolution of this proposal, reporting on my past four years of teacher education practice as I try to act on my own suggestions to this end and produce what I am calling a "sensory curriculum" for social justice teacher education.

The chapter proceeds as follows. In the next section, I describe my neo-materialist theoretical framework, defining assemblage and threshold, or the intensive, sensate edge of an assemblage where it threatens to unbecome itself and become other. I then describe my study's methodology for locating the intensive thresholds of the SJTE-assemblage in real-time and feeling for what happens when SJTE threatens to unbecome: when local events threaten to move beyond what is thinkable as "social justice teacher education" or what "social justice teacher educators" can do or say without losing this attribution. In order to situate the teaching practices that are the center of this chapter, I briefly describe my dissertation findings, focusing on what they suggest for a SJTE practice that mobilizes affect in order to prepare teachers to welcome a social difference that is not stable or static: one that they cannot yet imagine. I suggest that to proceed as though SJTE is static and generalizable is to presume that the things that SJTE attends to—forms and effects of social difference—are similarly static and generalizable. In my view, a more ethical presumption is that everything we offer teacher candidates will necessarily fall apart given the in-motion quality of social difference. The thing to do, then, is to prepare them as best as we can to expect, encounter and welcome this motion as the work of doing justice. The penultimate section focuses on my own teaching practice and its beginnings of a "sensory curriculum" for SJTE that tries, partially and provisionally, to do just that.

THEORY: DIPPING INTO ASSEMBLAGES

Theories of *assemblage*, a concept originating in the ontological collaborations of Gilles Deleuze and Félix Guattari (1987, 1996, 2004), and indebted in its later elaborations to many proponents of neo-materialism, are central to the arguments in this chapter. As a theoretical movement, neo-materialism seeks to remove Enlightenment humanism and human subjects from our self-installed position at the center of all things. The movement takes its bearings from philosophers like, as above, Gilles Deleuze and Felix Guattari, but also from feminist theorists like Rosi Braidotti, Elizabeth Grosz, and Claire Colebrook, Karen Barad and Donna Haraway. The neo-materialist turn involves locating agency in matter or substance and the processes by which it is organized, and not only in the actions of self-knowing human subjects. Rather, neo-materialists hold that matter—including that which composes the human body—acts and is acted upon in ways that precede or altogether exceed the human subject's knowledge. In other words, we cannot isolate significance to the moment when the human becomes able to narrate (whether for the other or the self) a feeling (this is how "I" feel) or perception (this is what "I" perceive). The never-narrated may be just as significant as that which we can say we know for sure. To this end, neo-materialists look to things that escape our perception, or that we can only know by the trace sensations left behind in their wake (Massumi, 2002). They also theorize the complex agency of matter itself as an actor (e.g., Chen, 2012) as opposed to matter as entities that only become significant when human subjects interact with them in some way.

Deleuze and Guattari's (1987) major vehicle for displacing human agency as the be-all and end-all of significance is the assemblage. For the purposes of this chapter,[1] I define assemblage as an ever-changing network of relations among human and non-human components, relations that are relentless (always forming), unpredictable, and non-hierarchical (i.e., rhizomatic—see Deleuze & Guattari, 1987; Martin & Kamberelis, 2013). Because of the ongoing, always-emergent nature of such relations, assemblages have no essential identity that transcends space and time. Instead, assemblages have properties that emerge when their components move about as they exercise their capacities. Unlike a static verifiable entity that post-positivism (see Lather, 2006) can pin down, locate outcomes for, and generalize across contexts, then, an assemblage continually changes in response to *local* conditions.

When conceptualized as an assemblage, SJTE *is* the aggregated effect of what its components *do* in everyday life. This is a theoretical move from examining linear and sequential connections between knowing *subjects* to a focus on the intertwined movements of connected *components*, of which humans happen to be but one type. DeLanda (2006) asserts that there is no linear causality ("same cause, same effect, always") in assemblages, troubling the attribution of an essential identity like "real SJTE" to a particular teacher education program or approach. SJTE's identity in its literature—as people who work to narrow various divides between privileged and oppressed groups of students for example—depends on a particular logic of linear causality: a greater number of particularly-oriented people doing particular things will lead to a necessarily more socially-just outcome. This cause and effect chain cannot be presumed within the ontological shift enacted by assemblage theory. From this perspective, linear causality cannot help us to definitively understand what SJTE *is* or *is not* because the SJTE-assemblage is only ever *becoming*.

Like linear causality, *internal* causality attributed to a single subject also fails in assemblage ontology because assemblage components never act in isolation. Things happen in assemblages because non-linear and external (situational) causality have produced a composite response to a provocation. In other words, a particular set of events occurs in a given instance and produces one of many possible responses. For DeLanda (2006), non-linear and external forms of causality are "defined by thresholds below or above which external causes fail to produce an effect" (p. 20). Instead of internal or linear causality, circumstances of *redundant* causality can create a context in which a component may be triggered but the entire assemblage may not respond. In the language of neo-materialisms, thinking with external causality means that individual component-level explanations are redundant when accounting for the emergent properties and capacities of an assemblage. Practically speaking, this means that it does not *matter* what "I meant" by my (in)action because I was always necessarily caught up with other components in producing a *material* event regardless of my own intent or even my awareness.

Assemblage ontology carries grave implications for agency or wakefulness as pivot points of social justice because a component never acts in isolation; rather, it is always affected by its relations to other components that include its own constituent parts and possibilities. A single person's (component's) actions—however highly-positioned they might be in a hierarchy—have only redundant causality such that I can never be said to have acted entirely on my own. At best, components including ourselves have a *composite* agency wherein "what I do" only actualizes because it can: because other components are actualizing capacities which enable this action, whether or not I am aware of those components or their capacities. For example, the capacity could be to only notice some things and not others or that I do not notice myself not noticing. Mechanisms of external causality therefore continually produce collective unintended consequences, even of actions that can be said to involve human agency.

Overall, then, human subjects can do things, but these things are not singular (i.e., done on one's own) nor any kind of determining factor in how things unfold. Composite agency is a useful notion for SJTE practitioners who often face an uphill pedagogical battle with students on the significance of intentionality—whether I did or didn't "mean it"—for determining harm and responsibility in instances of things like racism and homophobia. Usefully, composite agency also troubles any sense that knowing what I did (and to whom) actually matters. However, these ideas are so ontologically alien to most of us that the best way to infuse them in teacher education might not be through language and reason—explaining assemblage theory, for example—but through corporeal, sensory experience, a point to which I return in the description of my pedagogy below.

Having established some implications of assemblage theory for causality and agency as per DeLanda (2006), I now turn to Jeffrey Bell's (2006) theory of assemblages as dynamic systems at the edge of chaos. Where DeLanda provides an understanding of how and from what assemblages are composed, as well as the role of the subject-as-component within them, Bell is helpful in understanding how assemblages emerge, remain and die (become unidentifiable). Bell takes up the Deleuzian argument that things are never what they are, definitively. This is a direct challenge to traditional (Western) metaphysics in which thing-identity or being reaches its fullest expression when stable identities emerge and remain unchanging such that they are "complete." The criteria for completion are often images or ideas of the perfection that is commonly but not always associated with divinity (but perhaps, in SJTE and allied pursuits, with "social justice" as a more perfect ordering of the world). In transcendental metaphysics, things are *either* perfect *or* they are not, and perfection is completion. In Deleuzian metaphysics, however, being is a both-and in that complex things (assemblages) are *both* complete *and* in process; there is no binary between things "all done" and things "on the way." To be complete is to be in process in an assemblage's own singular way.

As such, Deleuze turned transcendental metaphysics on its head by suggesting that there *is* something eternal that exceeds being, but it is not a static ideal (i.e., divinity or "social justice"). What exceeds being is the both-and process of things continually changing and becoming. Bell (2006) characterizes assemblages as "dynamic systems" because they are always in motion, and describes them as "at the edge of chaos" because they work toward a plateau in between two kinds of death, chaos and cosmos.[2] Bell refers to this motion between the two extremes as "chaosmos." All dynamic systems navigate the two poles of chaosmos without succumbing to either cosmos-stasis through an excess of order or succumbing to chaos-collapse through meaningless proliferation. The cosmotic assemblage dies (ceases to be identifiable) because it resists crucial adaptation to a continuously becoming world, and the chaotic assemblage dies because it loses all consistency. To survive, assemblages must be affected by events without calcifying in resistance or allowing events to carry everything away. Completeness is not, therefore, a matter of reaching the end of a trajectory or the pinnacle of development, but of continually moving, where all movement is between the two poles. A *plateau* is the assemblage's achievement: where it has achieved sufficient consistency to create in sustainable ways but not enough to become static. A plateau is never a final resting place or stable signifier; it is rather the middling, back-and-forth journey between chaos and cosmos.

Sustainability, not radical change, is the politic implied by Deleuzo-Guattarian (1987) assemblage theory, hence their axiomatic quotation: "[staying] stratified—organized, signified, subjected—is not the worst that can happen; the worst that can happen is if you throw the strata into demented or suicidal collapse which brings them back down on us heavier than ever" (p. 161). From this perspective, the best, most life-producing change happens by degrees and through experimentation. Social justice educators and advocates, seeking sustainable change (as I do) through gradual consciousness-raising, coalition-building and consensual resource redistribution, are in a way acting from an implicit assemblage ontology. The pedagogy described in the next section is an expression of this gradualness.

Importantly, the continual becoming of an assemblage *is what the assemblage is*: how it responds to provocations and stimuli *is* its identity. In other words, an assemblage *is what it does* in order to stay malleable-enough and stable-enough while responding to stimuli, which are often figured as lines or flows of desire, energy, or intensity (DeLanda, 2006; Deleuze & Guattari, 1987). My dissertation study was an effort to track what happens when the SJTE-assemblage responds, in real-time, to a stimulus at its thresholds; stimuli are flows of affect, force, or desire (often referred to as "lines" in Deleuzian conversations). Three Deleuzian keywords help us to understand what can happen at an assemblage threshold: territorialization, deterritorialization, both gradual, and re-territorialization, which is swift and traumatic. My own addition is using the term "intervention" (as in, a territorializing intervention, for example) to describe what happens when an assemblage responds to provocation(s).

Each of the three processes does something to a line of force, as above, but are differentiated by their affective qualities: speed, force, volume, pitch, and so forth. In my fieldwork at SJTE-related conferences and conversations with practitioners, I identified three overarching types of interventions: (a) territorializing interventions where a line *gradually yet consistently* became rigidly segmented, chopped up, and slowed down through a "gentle suffocation;" (b) re-territorializing interventions where wild lines of flight were blocked and snuffed out in a *swift* "smack-down"; and (c) very slow deterritorializing interventions that wavered back and forth, eventually producing *sustainable* change in the local SJTE-assemblage (Airton, 2014).

METHODOLOGY AND FINDINGS: FROM ASSEMBLAGE TO AFFECT

My methodology for tracking SJTE's emergent thresholds and related interventions took place on the surface of the field's everyday life: in innumerable conversations, encounters and spaces shared briefly with shifting constellations of SJTE practitioners (teacher educators). In these moments, I mapped the unfolding experience of being "caught up" in the SJTE-assemblage as something "directly compelling" (Stewart, 2007, p. 3). As such, my dissertation insists that an assemblage can be studied on the visceral plane of *affect*, or, that affect is the means by which one's component-status in assemblages becomes apparent in everyday life. Following Brian Massumi (1987, 2002), I define *affect* as sensation or intensity that precedes our individual and idiosyncratic self-awareness, which is why we use the term "prepersonal" to describe affect as something prior to what is personal, or directly about the subject (Massumi, 1987). For Massumi (2002), affect is *unqualified* intensity because we are affected long before we can narrate intensity into emotions proper to ourselves as subjects. Or, the qualified personal experience that we call "emotion" is not the first thing that happens. Rather, affect precedes the (personal) experience entrenched through narration, or, as Claire Colebrook (2002) argues, " 'affect' is what happens to us when we feel an event" and is not "the meaning of an experience but the response it prompts" (p. xix). Lastly, affect is a fleetingness of *sensation* through which we can sense (then perhaps narrate later on) that something has happened because it has moved on and moved through us (Massumi, 2002). This change is what the subject—whether researcher or teacher—can apprehend, belatedly, through sensation. In its capacity as a conduit and impressionable surface for autonomous, circulating affect-as-sensation, the body apprehends much more and prior to the individual subject.

My methodological (and, as we shall see, pedagogical) argument is that assemblages make sensory landfall directly in the lives and on the bodies of their human (and non-human) components as affects; in this way, I argue that assemblages can be materially apparent despite their diffusion and decentered agency. Attuning one's self to rises and falls in affective intensity as the assemblage moves around and nears its thresholds is one way to study things that precede and exceed the words with which subjects narrate "my feelings" or "my intentions." Through variations in intensity registered in and as sensation, we can come to sense when the assemblage (in which we are one caught-up component) has come to a threshold.

The following is one possible brief description of what using affect to map assemblage thresholds can "look like" as a methodology. At conferences, my multi-sensory fieldwork involved using my eyes and ears but moreover my own body as a barometer of sensation—tensions, hunches, burnings, oscillations of alertness, and boredom—to follow affective intensities. At times I would pause and "take the pulse" of a room. This involved looking and feeling for how things were going, and how fast, how loud, how sudden, attentions to things like: comings/goings, modes and degrees of attentiveness, nods, vocalizations, twitches, snacking, drinking, program flipping, looking around, fidgeting, and so forth, relative to what was "happening" at the time. My scare quotes around "happening" are intended to convey that "what happened" was not limited to a speaker's presentation, for example, but included all other movements and utterances before, within and after a session's official timeframe. When the human subject's agency and intentionality are decentered, we can come to understand The Event as someone getting up and leaving a room, even if "The Event" itself—that is, the reason for being there—is a keynote. The Event can actually be everything we thought would be a non-event.

In conversations with practitioners, I would ask broad, open questions about their teaching, encouraging both speculation and generalization. My questions were an effort to stage the threshold of what "social justice teacher education" feels like: what is authentic and good, not just good-enough or insufficiently XYZ to be SJTE. I would directly pressure the "sore spots" of SJTE like evidence (my own research problem) and impostors. For example, I often asked whether practitioner intention or effect determines something to be "real SJTE." Importantly, I did not separate myself as "the interviewer" but rather tracked rises and falls in sensation to track affective intensities in each conversation between SJTE practitioners (including me).

Using this sensory methodological approach in both conferences and conversations, I identified and tracked all three kinds of intervention described in the previous section. However, the key finding of my dissertation came from tracking *de*territorializing interventions. These interventions, I found, exemplified Deleuzian political possibilities as

SJTE practitioners embraced our field's own contradictions, sore spots, and inconsistencies, even uttering words or questions otherwise anathema to "SJTE people" but present and pressing, none the less. In these uncertain and creative moments, SJTE became other in response to emerging local conditions, expressing a flexibility in SJTE that is absent from most of the field's defining literature. Rather, I argued, SJTE can tolerate local and partial iterations of itself which do not use "our language" but still do the work of social-justice-in-action. Pivotally, "the work" is tolerating and becoming open to our own and others' difference even from the most cherished foundations we have come to rest on and codify into language until they no longer keep up with everyday life (cosmos). There may be no one "real SJTE," clear and coherent, that unites us all across contexts.

Furthermore, by tracking any instances of talk about what happens when SJTE seems like it is 'going well' in the teacher education classroom, I developed a composite description of SJTE's *affective craft*. This craft entails acting pedagogically within an assemblage ontology and thereby centering things beyond our own control, with all that this implies for agency and subjectivity; it means teaching from the understanding that, to echo Lauren Berlant (2011), we and our students are non-sovereign. Regardless of what it looks or feels like in a particular local context, the craft of SJTE involves becoming attuned to the sensory barometer of one's own classroom and finding ways to increase or decrease affective intensity in the moment in order to produce the possibility of sustainable change or learning. Doing "good SJTE" in real-time is not ensuring that our students will be able to "teach for social justice," but modulating classroom affect to produce a plateau where slow, gradual and sustainable change can take place in our students' capacities to welcome difference. This modulation can even require us to provoke forms of student *resistance*, whether chaotic (loud, strident, interjecting) or cosmotic (quiet, withdrawn, stifling), in order to move a classroom-assemblage back to the productive middle where change emerge and stabilize.

I argue that, for teachers committed to making the world less harmful toward and more welcoming of social difference—both what is presently held to be different and the difference-to-come—this craft is as politically and ethically significant as the mastery of SJTE's (language-based) conceptual archive. As a field, SJTE practitioners should bring this expertise out of the ether of tacit contributions and directly into our work with teacher candidates. In addition to arguing that this affective craft should be *explicitly* exercised in the teacher education classroom, I also contend that it can and should be cultivated in our teacher candidates.

PEDAGOGY: MODULATING AFFECT, PRODUCING SENSORY CURRICULUM

How might SJTE practitioners exercise our affective craft in the classroom? What kind of SJTE pedagogy might foster our students' capacity for openness to unknowable social difference, instead of only moving along preexisting gridlines (Massumi, 2002)? In what follows, I describe a pedagogy that I am developing for this purpose. The text below is a composite of several first classes in SJTE courses that I have taught over the past five years, narrated together as a single moment in time. The pedagogies that I describe—the Awkward Moment and the Follow-Your-Gut Essay—are necessarily provisional attempts to *do something* as teacher but from a non-sovereign starting place: to produce threshold moments where my students can sense, tolerate and hopefully begin to act from the inevitability of an assemblage social field where their sovereign intentionality does not, literally, matter.

Part 1: The Awkward Moment

The room is set up in a fairly conventional way with pods of tables and chairs, and an introductory slide is on the screen bearing the course title and my name. In other words, there is no way the students can doubt that they are in the right place. Not only is this a classroom, but it is clearly marked as one in which I am their teacher. I circulate as students enter, greeting them in a friendly way and offering small talk here and there, working to ensure that as many students as possible have either interacted with me in a casual way or seen this happen before I formally begin the lesson. In other words, I seek to produce and stabilize the expectation of an easygoing professor with a sense of humor.

When all (or most) students have arrived and found a seat, I take up an archetypal teacher position in the very front of the room, blocking the projection screen to indicate that my presence should now take precedence over all other stimuli including my own slides. Mobilizing teacher-form and teacher-content, I call them to order in a clear and authoritative voice: "hello everyone! Let's get started now." There is no room for ambiguity; class has now begun. Thirty-odd young adults begin to dial down their movements and conversations as the ambient noise recedes.

They wait, but I do not speak. Instead, I move my eyes over them with an easy smile, making brief eye contact with students in no discernible pattern and holding my body in an alert yet relaxed position in front of them. They become collectively more still and more quiet by degrees, as if to note a collective deficiency: they must be insufficiently ready for me to proceed.

By now, there is virtually no sound or movement in the room. And still, I do not speak nor give them direction of any kind. The thing they have done together to produce my speech has not worked. And so, without consultation or conversation, the student-body tries something else. At first, there is a quivering around the edges, like muscle fatigue. From absolute stillness of movement come shiftings-around in seats, an uncrossing of knees or ankles. Many break their gaze on me to scan their peripheral vision. Scanning gradually becomes engagement with each other. Initially tentative and then more deliberate eye contact succumbs to full-blown communication as they engage in an array of facial expressions, conveying everything from anxiety to disbelief to mirth. Their asked but unspoken questions: is this professor for real? What is happening? What kind of course is this? There is giggling, then laughter, then outright speech as some students whisper and then begin asking aloud these questions of each other.

And still I do not speak.

And then, a (territorializing) threshold: a student says something, out loud, *to me*. This first talker offers a greeting or a question. I count a few seconds—long enough to dial up the intensity, nameable as an anxiety that even this last ditch effort will not produce what they desire—and then respond in an open and kindly way, either by returning the greeting or answering the question. Back from the brink, we are becoming-classroom once again, and I becoming-teacher.

With my reply, the surface tension breaks: the students move and speak freely, exhaling and sighing in relief. This was incredibly taxing and uncomfortable. *Awkward.* I join them in the exhales and sighs, moving my body around the front of the classroom as I begin to ask some debrief questions, starting with the most simple: what just happened? Chalk in hand, I write their responses on the blackboard in order to build back some trust that I will be their teacher. At first, they only talk about my behavior: that I did not speak or move very much, that I did not begin class. With prompting, they begin to talk about their own behavior but firmly in a register of "we" and "our." It is as if their own actions are invisible to them as they focus on the collective action of the whole. I then focus on the first talker: why did you speak? Why did you say what you said? Unknowingly recognizing their only-ever composite agency, this student is often unable to identify a distinct decision that they made, whether to speak at all or what to say. It just happened. I then ask the others how they felt at that moment: were they grateful to the first talker? I ask them to imagine what would happen if even this direct address had not produced my response. Would there have been a confrontation? Would they have left? These potentials are virtually bodied-forth in still more giggles, shiftings-around and similar micromovements that index the chaos kept at bay.

At this point, I usually introduce five terms that we will use throughout the remainder of the course to explore topics related to social difference in education. While I do not offer citation, I explain that I am defining these terms in the interdisciplinary sense in which they have come to be used by queer theorists over the past few decades:[3]

- norm (n.)—unapparent (i.e., invisible) standard that guides behavior
- normative (adj.)—conforms with the norm
- non-normative (adj.)—does not conform with the norm
- normalization (n.)—process through which X becomes normative
- normalize (v.)—to produce normalization

Once I have defined these terms and assessed whether their relationship is broadly understood, I support the students in using these terms to describe the event that I just worked to produce in our class. First, I ask a question-in-disguise about assemblage thresholds: *what actions were non-normative*? They are readily able to identify my own behavior as non-normative: that I was not teacher-enough. By inverting their descriptions of what I did *not* do, I sketch our emergent definition of "teacher" on the board: directs students in what they should be doing, is responsive to students, makes students comfortable. We discuss: is it necessarily the teacher's job to make students comfortable? Do their philosophies of teaching match the emergent definition they produced?

Our definition anticipates my follow-up question: *what was the unapparent norm being transgressed?* I observe that norms become apparent to us when they are on the verge of being transgressed, or when they are ruptured altogether. Because my behavior transgressed a norm (or, neared a threshold), that norm became apparent, but it is always actively structuring our engagement with each other even as we do not notice it doing so. My third debrief question is the most important: *what actions were normalizing* (or, what kind of intervention took place at the threshold)? In their responses, students begin to implicate themselves in the process which they will come to recognize as the micropolitical mechanism for perpetuating *inter alia* whiteness, heteronormativity, settler-colonialism and able-bodiedness as we proceed through the course. Pivotally, they identify their own participation in normalization—in trying to push me toward a normative performance of teacher and teaching—as something collective: without consciousness or intentionality on their part. Their bodies were caught up in actions all the way from their initial stillness/quietness to subtle movement to eye contact to facial expressions to giggles to laughter to whispers to speech to—at long last—someone speaking to me, directly, and still unable to recall a clear moment of decision making. Our curriculum is the sensory memory of their own unwitting participation.

Having begun to sense and now recognize their implicit participation in the process by which norms stabilized and emerge over and over again, the students now prepare for the same sort of fieldwork that I myself enacted in completing my dissertation research: to take this sensory memory into the streets and their everyday lives. The culmination of this field work is the Follow-Your-Gut Essay.

Part 2: The Follow-Your-Gut Essay

The Follow-Your-Gut Essay (the Essay, going forward) is a paper with three parts that revolves around what I call a "gut event" in students' everyday lives as they move about in public space. In diverse urban settings, the best place to do their field work is public transit. And so, with our above Awkward Moment as an affective template (in form not content), I instruct them to stay alert on their daily commute for any instance of the following:

- something that causes them to perform a double-take;
- something that they cannot wait to tell someone else about later on;
- or something that they wish their friend, and so forth, was also there to see.

Key here is that their body, affected and affecting, takes the lead. You cannot consciously seek out your gut event, I tell them. Rather, it will find you. Because sensation is fleeting (Massumi, 2002), they will only know that an event has transpired when it is already receding into the past: when they feel their head turning to look again, or when they catch themselves in the act of taking a photo, texting a friend or telling the story later on. Once they have belatedly registered their bodies being caught up in a collective intervention (the event), I instruct them to write with as much detail about what was taking place around them: who, what (before, during, and after), where, when, and a description of how their body reacted. In just one week, they usually have several gut events to choose from.

For the first component of the Essay, they select one event and write up their field notes into an evocative narrative. One criterion is that the reader must be able to feel our way into the event, which they are to privilege over verbatim representation (see Stewart, 2007). I expect vivid description of their own and others' actions, including those of the focal point person (if applicable) and others in the vicinity, as well how they felt. They are also invited to extend themselves into hypotheticals and feel their potential:

what might have happened if XYZ had happened next, for example, or if the focal point person (if applicable) had appeared otherwise?

The second and third components are more reflective in nature. Students are first instructed to "look inward," or, to take accountability for being seized by the event; instead of resting with "anyone would think that was weird, out of place, etc." they must answer the question: why did this event stand out to *me*, in particular? What issues were raised by the event, and what in their own histories and experiences has also connected to those issues? How are they socially positioned in relation to the others caught up in its unfolding? After taking this "inward" accountability, the students are instructed to "look outward," or, to explore others' thinking and writing on the issues raised by the event. These sources can take any form, be they conversations had or overheard, sub-Reddits, Tweets, research papers, magazine articles, blog posts, TV shows, or films. The students give a brief account of these other perspectives, and then discuss them alongside their event. In the Essay's conclusion, they share implications for their future practice as teachers. What have they learned about themselves and what their non-sovereign body does, unwittingly, that they can take with them into the classroom?

Having evaluated many other reflective assignments in teacher education courses about social justice, diversity and/or equity, I am struck by the local, micropolitical specificity invited and perhaps enabled by the Essay. With all identifying details removed, here is a brief sample of what some students have written about:

- After being startled by a feminine-presenting "cross-dresser" while scavenging for firewood in an urban ravine and immediately crafting witty text messages about the encounter, a straight cis-gender male student critiques his use of humor as a tool of gender normalization in many areas of his life, including as a teacher.
- While adopting a kitten, a vegan student becomes angry when another shelter visitor seeks confirmation that her own kitten can be brought back if need be, and then explores how her social class may enable her staunch animal rights politics.
- A Chinese immigrant student recounts an event which triggered her own Islamophobia and traces it to scary bedtime stories about Uighurs (a Muslim minority group in China) used to frighten young children into good behavior.
- After strong disgust at the sight of someone feeding pigeons, a student develops a critique of the human-animal divide based on her own experiences of racialization.

- A split-second double take at a punk on the subway prompts a student to interrogate her immigrant family's overriding preoccupation with dressing to appear affluent, at all times and in all places, without exception.
- After being asked by a racialized bus driver for her transfer and seeing another white passenger explode in a racist tirade over same, a white student considers how her own annoyance could have been read as (and, moreover, was produced as) an expression of white privilege.

In each admittedly partial example, sensation leads a student into an achingly micropolitical reckoning with their non-sovereignty. Critically, each student refuses recourse to mastery discourse: to any claim that they control how they affect or are affected in everyday life. All is in-process, including progressive bona fides (vegetarianism, animal rights politics) that can so often shield us from reproach, placing us unstintingly on some "correct side" of grand social justice struggle. Consciousness and intentionality cease to determine a student's role in everyday low-level racisms and transphobias. Linearities of meaning dissipate, yielding rhizomatic (Deleuze & Guattari, 1987) connections between, for example, real-time punk aesthetics and the visceral residue of immigrant respectability. Each event is something that *undeniably happened*, in the immediate past tense, and the student is asked to consider it from the visceral, sensory knowledge that something unfolded prior to and beyond their agency: something that matters perhaps even more so because it cannot be subjectively controlled.

Many familiar and SJTE-friendly pedagogies of consciousness-raising ask students to own up to their own complicity in oppression after learning the history and proper application of these terms. Conversely, the Awkward Moment and the Follow Your Gut Essay reverse the timeline: first we register our undeniable caught-up complicity in things larger and far more complex than ourselves, and then we reflect. What happens after that cannot be known in advance, including whether this "reflection" (precise meaning here unknown) could ever be something like readiness to practice social justice education, recalling my discussion of SJTE's outcome and evidence problems that began this chapter. And although the Awkward Moment and the Follow Your Gut Essay do lean on my own agency as teacher educator, they are structured from the recognition that the teacher's agency is only ever compromised, composite and ultimately non-sovereign.

CONCLUSION: LEARNING TO PAUSE

This two-part sensory curriculum for social justice teacher education is my current answer to two questions arising out of my dissertation: first, when working with beginning teachers, how can we avoid circumscribing social difference via our curriculum resources, an unintended consequence of needing objects for students to engage with before they have field data of their own? Any static representations of "racism," "homophobia," and so forth, might only prepare them to encounter the representation, and not things emerging otherwise where they come to practice. This problem inspired both the Moment (as well as similar ways in which I labor to produce threshold events in the course of my teaching) and the Essay. My second question: how might we prepare teachers with the skills to welcome social difference as it emerges in real-time, instead of being caught up in normalization and/as re-territorialization before they can recognize an event? My provisional strategy is to cultivate teachers' capacity to register sensation—their component status within multiple, shifting assemblages—and then, quite simply, pause: pause, and then be slowly, incrementally and always-partially guided by their senses in thinking and, moreover, feeling through the escaping intensity.

In my Deleuzo-Guattarian (1987) rendering, welcoming difference demands the visceral ability to do something like "go with the flow" of a particular context or encounter as it unfolds, without seeking to control it and without recourse to claims about our intentionality in so doing. This is part of pausing when we sense the welling-up of intensity as someone or something arrives (e.g., onto our bus or streetcar) to loosen our a priori expectations, which are often things never narrated (which implies absolutely nothing about their power or significance). My hope is that, over time, the pause can slow normalization and/as re-territorialization: that through the provisional recognition of their non-sovereignty, students can enable more by doing less.

I use derivatives of "norm" in a highly processual way to cue students into how the unthought norm is never static. It is actually always being produced, including via their own non-sovereign participation: becoming-normal, always in-process, produced and producing dynamic states of normativity. After the pause comes, perhaps, reflection: what must the student engage with, expose themselves to, or think more about in order to soften (but never prevent) the likelihood of their being caught up in this way in the future? Critically, the pause happens prior to the privilege confessional and its paradox: that the reasons why we might expect particular things of the other do not actually matter in the moment when the expectation is acted out against our will. Even our most changed intentions do not matter, in the sense of the material. Intentionality is too late to the party, where sensation has already erupted onto the scene and swept us along in a tide of normalization: of shutting out and shutting down the percolating flow of the sustainably new. Helping teacher candidates learn to "get out ahead" of themselves and deprioritize their good intentions is, I argue, helping them to develop their own affective craft.

At the core of my research and teaching is this tenet: that paying attention to and learning from our own non-sovereign responses to social difference and/as the non-normative can develop the capacity to *actually enact* a relation to the other which is open to and not foreclosing of difference, both the first time and every time thereafter. This is a critical starting place for preparing teachers to create a classroom that welcomes and fosters forms of difference that, first, we cannot yet imagine but that will someday walk through their classroom doors, and second, that are already present and yet unrecognizable. To create an open space for students and ourselves as teachers to emerge otherwise, and not to normalize that difference into stasis. This, in my view, is the craft of social justice teachers and teacher educators alike.

NOTES

1. For my discussion of assemblages, I am indebted to Manuel DeLanda (2006) and Jeffrey Bell (2006) (see Airton, 2014 for a complete discussion of each one's assemblage theory and how I relate them to each other).
2. Significantly, this word does not here relate to "the cosmos" in the sense of outer space and celestial bodies.
3. In addition to assemblage theory and affect theory, queer theory is another touchstone of my research and teaching. In the next and last section, I will further explain my use of these terms and how they relate to the theoretical framework I have laid out in the preceding sections. Elsewhere, I have begun to engage the connections between Deleuzian metaphysics and queer theory (see Airton, 2013).

REFERENCES

Ahmed, S. (2012). *On being included: Racism and diversity in institutional life*. Durham, NC: Duke University Press.

Airton, L. (2013). Leave "those kids" alone: On the conflation of school homophobia and suffering queers. *Curriculum Inquiry, 43*(5), 531–562. doi:10.1111/curi.12031

Airton, L. (2014). *Be(coming) the change you want to see in the world: Social justice teacher education as affective craft* (Unpublished doctoral dissertation). York University, Toronto ON. Retrieved from https://yorkspace.library.yorku.ca/xmlui/bitstream/handle/10315/28286/Airton_Lee_JE_2014_PhD.pdf?sequence=2

Bell, J. A. (2006). *Philosophy at the edge of chaos: Gilles Deleuze and the philosophy of difference*. Toronto, ON: University of Toronto Press.

Berlant, L. (2011). *Cruel optimism*. Durham, NC: Duke University Press.

Chen, M. Y. (2012). *Animacies: Biopolitics, racial mattering, and queer affect*. Durham, NC: Duke University Press.

Cochran-Smith, M., Barnatt, J., Lahann, R., Shakman, K., & Terrell, D. (2009). Teacher education for social justice: Critiquing the critiques. In W. Ayers, T. Quinn, & D. Stovall (Eds.), *The handbook of social justice in education* (pp. 625–639). London, England: Taylor & Francis.

Cochran-Smith, M., Davis, D., & Fries, K. (2004). Multicultural teacher education: Research, practice, and policy. In J. A. Banks & C. A. M. Banks (Eds.), *Handbook of research on multicultural education* (2nd ed., pp. 931–975). San Francisco, CA: Jossey-Bass.

Colebrook, C. (2002). *Gilles Deleuze*. New York, NY: Routledge.

DeLanda, M. (2006). *A new philosophy of society: Assemblage theory and social complexity*. London, England: Continuum.

Deleuze, G., & Guattari, F. (1987). *A thousand plateaus: Capitalism and schizophrenia*. (B. Massumi, Trans.) (1st ed.). Minneapolis, MN: University of Minnesota Press.

Deleuze, G., & Guattari, F. (1996). *What is philosophy?* (H. Tomlinson & G. Burchell, Trans.). New York, NY: Columbia University Press.

Deleuze, G., & Guattari, F. (2004). *Anti-Oedipus: Capitalism and schizophrenia* (R. Hurley, M. Seem, & H. R. Lane, Trans.). London, England: Continuum.

Dover, A. G. (2009). Teaching for social justice and K–12 student outcomes: A conceptual framework and research review. *Equity & Excellence in Education, 42*(4), 506–524. doi:10.1080/10665680903196339

Gorski, P. C. (2010). The scholarship informing the practice: Multicultural teacher education philosophy and practice in the US. *International Journal of Multicultural Education, 12*(2), 1–22.

Grant, C. A., & Secada, W. (1990). Preparing teachers for diversity. In W. Houston, M. Haberman, & J. Sikula (Eds.), *Handbook of research on teacher education* (pp. 403–422). New York, NY: Macmillan.

Hollins, E. R., & Guzman, M. T. (2005). Research on preparing teachers for diverse populations. In M. Cochran-Smith & K. M. Zeichner (Eds.), *Studying teacher education: The report of the AERA Panel on Research and Teacher Education* (pp. 477–541). New York, NY: Routledge.

Ladson-Billings, G. (1995). Multicultural teacher education: Research, practice, and policy. In J. Banks & C. A. McGee Banks (Eds.), *Handbook of research on multicultural education* (pp. 747–759). San Francisco, CA: Jossey-Bass.

Lather, P. (2006). Paradigm proliferation as a good thing to think with: Teaching research in education as a wild profusion. *International Journal of Qualitative Studies in Education, 19*(1), 35–57.

Lather, P. (2013). Methodology-21: What do we do in the afterward? *International Journal of Qualitative Studies in Education, 26*(6), 634–645.

Lather, P., & St. Pierre, E. A. (2013). Post-qualitative research. *International Journal of Qualitative Studies in Education, 26*(6), 629–633. doi:10.1080/09518398.2013.788752

Martin, A. D., & Kamberelis, G. (2013). Mapping not tracing: Qualitative educational research with political teeth. *International Journal of Qualitative Studies in Education, 26*(6), 668–679. doi:10.1080/09518398.2013.788756

Massumi, B. (1987). Translator's foreword: Pleasures of philosophy. In B. Massumi (Trans.), G. Deleuze & F. Guattari, (Eds.), *A thousand plateaus: Capitalism and schizophrenia* (pp. ix–xvi). New York, NY: Continuum.

Massumi, B. (2002). *Parables for the virtual: Movement, affect, sensation*. Durham, NC: Duke University Press.

Mazzei, L. A. (2004). Silent listenings: Deconstructive practices in discourse-based research. *Educational Researcher, 33*(2), 26–34.

Mazzei, L. A. (2009). An impossibly full voice. In A. Y. Jackson & L. A. Mazzei (Eds.), *Voice in qualitative inquiry: Challenging conventional, interpretive, and critical conceptions in qualitative research* (pp. 45–75). New York, NY: Routledge.

St. Pierre, E. A. (2013). The posts continue: Becoming. *International Journal of Qualitative Studies in Education, 26*(6), 646–67.

Stewart, K. (2007). *Ordinary affects*. Durham, NC: Duke University Press.

Villegas, A. M., & Lucas, T. (2002). *Educating culturally responsive teachers: A coherent approach*. Albany, NY: State University of New York Press.

Zeichner, K. M. (2009). *Teacher education and the struggle for social justice*. New York, NY: Routledge.

CHAPTER 4

WAR OF THE HALF-BREEDS

Communities of Color as a Resistant Response to Raced and Racist Education in the Midwest

Boni Wozolek
Loyola University Maryland

"Like I said, we are going to start a war—of the half-breeds—and we are going to take over that way, you know, everyone realizes we are all the same, you know. It's not just.... It's just like that for a lot of kids.... It's messed up. When we say 'war of the half-breeds' or whatever, it's just a little joke but in all reality, it's based off of that and... I don't think it would be just white and black people. I think it would be every race basically on the planet ... saying ... I don't want to spend my life being a color, you know?"

Throughout this chapter, there are QR codes linked to sound files of participants in this study. Although you can understand the general ideas without them, the arguments made throughout require sounds to be heard as they are placed in the chapter. Should the QR codes not function, each code has a footnote with a link that can be used to hear the files. The first file can be heard at: bit.ly/half-breeds1

Sensuous Curriculum:
Politics and the Senses in Education, pp. 67–83

This is a story about how a small group of male students of color resisted the places in their high school that were designed against their ways of being, as well as the spaces of whiteness that intentionally maintained self-fulfilling prophesies of failure for students of color. Their story, centered on questions of race and schooling, is certainly not new. Iterations of this narrative have been told across time (e.g., Cooper, 1892; Bethune, 1938; Rist, 1973; Winfield, 2007), gender (e.g., Gordon, 1993; Lorde, 1984; Woodson, 1933), and disciplines (e.g., DuBois, 1903; Heath, 1983; hooks, 1994; Jackson, 1968). For example, ethnographic accounts document the multiple ways marginalized student populations resist systems of oppression in schooling (Page, 1991; Tatum, 2003; Willis, 1977). In so doing, they serve not only as a backdrop to this chapter but stand as significant illustrations of the iterations and recursions across historical and contemporary contexts that inform students' lived experiences in schools.

Although racialized and racist systems of schooling are well documented, this chapter attends to the encounters in, between, and on bodies as they exist as everyday affects of oppression in schools. Attending to racism-as-affect requires attention to the often hard-to-name but indelibly-felt-and-known school encounters that both undergird and permeate daily experiences and ontologies for students of color. A lack of explicit attention to affect theory and studies of schooling often inadvertently and unintentionally perpetuate conceptualizations of race and schools as places where racism impacts students of color intellectually and emotionally, yet somehow travels only through intellectual exchanges. In short, what is being raised here is specifically a question of intention (as racism is often purposely constructed) and attention (as those being racist often do not attend to how their actions affect the victim). Any iteration of a racist event is therefore as much about emotional impacts as they slam into the people that are its targets as it regards the intellectual exchange and sociocultural contexts that engender such possibilities.

The narrative in this chapter focuses on racism-as-affect in schools as a means to unpack lines of power, privilege, and intention that impacted students in their daily lives at school. I begin by arguing that identifying racism-as-affect is a significant means for analyzing oppressive events that students of color experience through schooling. Next, I present a counter-narrative from a one-year ethnographic study with 17 young men of color at a large, suburban high school in the Midwest. Finally, I conclude this chapter by analyzing how my findings from this study resonate with long-standing dialogues on race and education in ways that further imbricate questions of affect and power for youth of color in and against systems in schooling.

SUCKER PUNCHES OF PRIVILEGE: AFFECT AND RACISM IN SCHOOLS

"We're like some type of majestic-ass bird ... and when you see us it's like doom's comin'"

File can be heard at: bit.ly/half-breeds2

From Cater G. Woodson's (1933) powerful text that explicates educational lynching as the process of teaching a student that "his black face is a curse and [that] his struggle to change his condition is hopeless" (p. 3), to Mary McLeod Bethune's (1939) depiction of the terror and humiliation of being denied civil liberties in school and society, racism is heard and felt through a multiplicity affective encounters and tensions. A central argument throughout the African American intellectual tradition is that racial oppression is not liminal but rather it hits, saturates and is ontologically toxic: Racism lands on bodies and permeates ways of being. In a contemporary context, as Black and Brown bodies are being attacked in the streets and imaginations are assaulted in classrooms, it is no surprise that renewed attention to scholars like James Baldwin and Frederick Douglass have broken the surface of mainstream American consciousness, especially during a political moment that has strong historical echoes of similar racial hostilities and oppressions.

To study dialogues throughout the African American intellectual tradition and its contemporary iterations (e.g., critical race theory, black feminisms, etc.) is to engage in affective knowledges. Theories of oppression with the physical and emotional narratives of being struck by racialized violence are continually imbricated in this stream of scholarship. For example, discourses on racial battle fatigue (RBF) tend to embody the nested layers of theory and lived experiences in the form of counternarratives (Mitchell, Fasching-Varner, Albert, & Allen, 2014; Smith, Yosso, & Solóranzo, 2006). Counternarratives often illustrate the sociocultural climate that engendered the event, the moment of experiencing racial hostilities, and the enduring effect on the victim's ways of knowing and being. This is important because RBF often unpacks the event and the effects. However, what is often missing from these powerful stories that resonate across contexts is the impact of such racist events on the body and being at the moment of experiencing the aggression.

For those who experience hatred and violence, the moment when racism impacts and affects your person is inevitable but somehow remains hard to name. Perhaps this is because the moment of impact is out of the victim's control, the focus of another's racist attentions and intentional malice—whether explicit or implied, moving from inside thoughts to affecting others requires intention. This is because racist acts are at once public and private. Similar to Kathleen Stewart's (2007) articulation of ordinary affects, racism-as-affect is felt as "public feelings that begin and end in broad circulation, but they're also the stuff that seemingly intimate lives are made of" (p. 2). Diverging from Stewart's more broad conceptualization of affects, which describes affect as potentially "a pleasure and a shock" (p. 2), here I am focusing on the perturbing, ontologically traumatic, socioculturally normalized trajectories of oppression that are expressed by one being through aggression and land as harm on and in the victim. Regardless of the frequency or familiarity with racist actions, patterns, systems, or institutions, as Bethune (1939) reminds us, being denied rights and possibilities through racisms is nonetheless a moment of "terror and humiliation" (p. 1). It is the sucker punch of privilege. No matter how often you've been hit, or your anticipation of the next swing, the emotional and physical impact passes through your whole body—there is an ontological difference between preparation and impact.

Racist confrontations are often discussed in terms of microaggressions in the literature on racial battle fatigue, a method specifically designed to capture the effects of encountering racialized hostilities (Smith, Yosso, & Solóranzo, 2006). Scholarship on microaggressions is significant because it simultaneously recognizes the varying degrees of racialized hostilities that impact people while describing the lasting effects of these actions. As I have argued elsewhere (Wozolek, 2014; Wozolek, Varndell, & Speer, 2015), although dialogue on how microaggressions function to continue oppression after the action has occurred is central to unpacking normalized racial hostilities, it can incidentally place aggressions on a false binary between the micro and the macro. To be clear, as I argued in my work on Queer Battle Fatigue (Wozolek, Varndell, & Speer, 2015), I am not equating physical brutalities to emotional and psychological violence. However, it is important to remember that even the most minor of microaggressions can have a deep and sustaining impact. Where racial battle fatigue is helpful in understanding the affective nodes of racism is in an underlying examination of the subtle everydayness of racist actions and how racisms have emotional and physical effects on the victims of these normalized aggressions. Racism-as-affect is therefore not only ontologically and epistemologically damaging but also affects one's physical self.

Sarah Ahmed (2010) writes that the stickiness of affect preserves connections between beings, bodies, and sociocultural norms and values. It is important to note that questions of agency are central to the study of affective encounters and that two significant layers of affects are the agencies of the aggressor and the person experiencing hostility. Although the original agency of affect came from a person, affect still operates after that person is gone—once it is in contact with a person, suck affect remains agential regardless of the aggressor's physical presence or absence. It is either a lingering affect from the person or it is an encounter that has collapsed layers—both historically and in the current context—so that the more you encounter, the deeper the impact. However, there are aspects of affect that hit bodies so deeply that they appear to move outside discussions of agency and culpability, moments when affect runs wild. And in those moments, we cannot help but to feel. When it's love and kindness that are affecting us, isn't it wonderful? But when hate and aggression deal blows to our being, there are moments when we are left with nothing but our affect.

As but one metaphorical example, consider the material combination of lead and water. Not only is lead dispersed through the water but, once ingested, it continues to damage the body. How lead interacts with water and bodies literally is a metaphorical parallel to the ways in which racism is enacted in sociocultural norms and values. The negative impacts of a direct encounter may not appear to be initially harmful, and be masked in apparent goodness of water, but will have lingering effects on those who must drink the water, as the ability to avoid contaminated water is a question of privilege. Avoiding lead tainted water means that one must have the necessary financial and cultural capital to live outside of zones with lead contaminated water, have the knowledge and money to consider testing, or the money for proper filtration.

The ability to serve others contaminated water without drinking it yourself is a question of agency as much as it is an expression of privilege, as is the ability to ignore those suffering from contaminated water. See, for example, the ongoing crisis in places like Flint, Michigan and the national response to urban victims. Racism-as-affect from this metaphorical understanding is not a question of lead being in the water but, rather, how much of the water one has to drink and whether or not you have the privilege of a filter. The lead, racism, is always in the water. Drinking water is a necessity to live. However, the ability to purchase, or being given, a filter to protect you from the carcinogens is a question of privilege. How one uses the filter, as an ally or accomplice for those who do not have filters, is a matter of agency.

Schools reflect sociocultural norms, values, policies, and practices, and, as such, often become a microcosm, and in many cases, concentrated versions of those sociocultural ideas.and ideals (Baldwin, 1962; Tatum, 2003; Woodson, 1933). For many marginalized students and groups, attending school is the emotional and physical equivalent of involuntarily swimming in and ingesting a distilled sample of lead-laden water (e.g., Rist, 1973; Winfield, 2007; Woodson, 1933). However, rather than attending to the multiple ways that racism affects students, many schools often focus on questions of agency on the part of the victim. For example, it is not unusual for students to be told, "You cannot control others but you can control how you react." While it is certainly true that students should be held accountable for their actions, little emphasis is placed on the affective tensions of everyday racism and their physical and emotional effect on students, both immediately and over time.

Although the aggressor (or "bully," to use the coded language of schools) is sometimes given punishment for their words, the penalty generally fits the crime for verbal assault. However, similar to the points raised by critical race scholars through constructs like racial battle fatigue, racism-as-affect centers on both the emotional and lasting physical effects of these hostilities. Resistance and resilience is therefore difficult and, as articulated in the narrative below, is a significant part of enacting agency within affective tensions and an unjust yet necessary part of survival to endure against racism as it spills into and hits young souls. In short, when racism is inserted, it becomes a spectral footprint of hate on one's way of being and knowing—resistance is but one way to stand up against the daily sucker punches of privilege.

GOING TO LOSE THE BATTLE: RESISTING THE SPACES AND PLACES OF SCHOOL

—*"What do you think I'm doing? … I'm walkin' to my locker. I'm not … robbin' anybody. Shooting anybody…"*

—*"I feel like we just can't trust the principals and some teachers … because they are going to try to flip something on you, get you in trouble in some way…. You report something bad that's happening and it somehow gets turned on you."*

File can be heard at: bit.ly/half-breeds3

As one of only 3 teachers of color at a Midwestern suburban high school with a student body of about 2,400, I often found myself moving quickly through the halls, working hard to go unnoticed by the largely white student and staff population. As I rushed to the copier one afternoon, located roughly a quarter mile walk from my classroom, I was stopped by a group of biracial male students who asked if I would be their leader. When I inquired about the activity I was to lead, I was informed by Darius [all proper nouns are pseudonyms], who I knew as one of the more boisterous young men in the group, that it was "for the war of the half-breeds, of course!" Smirking, he continued, "You're our only half-breed teacher, right? So, we need a leader. Wanna help?" I looked around and noted that the group was predominantly biracial and all male. I asked where the girls were and they pointed down the hall to a small group of young women of color. Marcus informed me that this part of the hall was called "Little Africa" by the students and staff alike as generations of students of color had congregated in the same area. He noted, however, that their group, called "The Crew," stayed at the bottom of the stairs because, on one hand, it "showed their position in life." Members of the group owned this physical and metaphorical space in similar ways how they claimed the "N" word as African American youth and, at the same time, they spoke about their sociocultural position with a degree of shame as they had been identified this way by their Anglo peers, teachers, and administration and such identification did not align with their personal identities. On the other hand, they also were clear that this location gave them a physical advantage as it intersected with a second hallway, giving them the opportunity to run down the hall or up the stairs when the administration decided to interrupt their daily assembly. I glanced over at the administrators who had their backs against the brick wall and were observing the flow of student traffic in the hallway at the end of the day.

That moment served as a catalyst for a year-long study investigating the ways that students of color negotiate the spaces and places of a predominantly white high school, a process that also became a scholarly journey of personal and professional vulnerability as I worked with the Crew in my dual roles as teacher and researcher. As Behar (1996) articulates, one of the central dilemmas of witnessing the horror that "looms gently in the memories that won't recede and so come pouring forth in the quiet" (p. 2) of, in this case the classrooms and corridors (for more on their intersections, see Metz, 1978), "as the storyteller opens her heart to the listener, recounting hurts that cut deep and raw into the gullies of the self, do you, the observer, switch on the tape recorder, keep pen in hand? But if you can't stop the horror, shouldn't you at least document it?" (Behar, 1996, p. 2). Often part of the fatigue we feel as researchers of color working with students of color is the emotional exhaustion of reliving our own horrors with racialized aggressions as we hear the stories of participants. This is important because despite the potentially targeted nature of affect between beings, it can often land on others not directly related to events (Gershon, 2013c). Racism as affect in the context of this study acted as the lead in my own drinking water as I existed as both the teacher and researcher of color. Being part of the systems of schooling, I had my own responsibility in both the disruption and recursion of the racism. Documenting the unstoppable horrors of racism in schooling, as Behar might argue, generated my own vulnerability to the context and simultaneous forms of resistance against it through recording the events.

Methodologically, as a narrative rooted in ethnographic traditions (Agar, 1996; Behar, 1996; Geertz, 1973; Gershon, 2009; Stoller, 1997), it was also a collaborative project that thought with this group of mostly seniors about questions of oppression and resistance to racism and schooling. Narratives in this study were collected through individual interviews, group interviews (both with and without the researcher present), and visual and auditory maps. As a part of contemporary critical geography and mapping practices (Gershon, 2013a; Harvey, 1973; Massey, 2005; Powell, 2010; Soja, 2010), students not only created maps of the spaces they felt were significant to the school but they also aided in the analysis process of these maps. It was through these multiple forms of conversation that I would quickly learn the multiple ways the Crew had used their time in school to develop a careful system through which they recruited and trained other students to deal with the pressures of schooling and marginalization. They felt, as Anthony explained during an interview, that "school already fucks you up, why shouldn't we have a way to make sure it doesn't fuck up everyone who doesn't fit in?"

Shaking Hands

As I rounded a corner and entered the stairwell, I heard voices rising up from the bottom of the stairwell. It was Marcus, Anthony, and a boy I did not recognize. I paused to eavesdrop on the conversation. It was one of those rare moments where I could listen quietly without my physical presence impeding conversation. I heard Marcus say, "Seriously? Goddamn, nigga…. That's what you call a handshake? Why don't you try it again?" This was followed quickly by the sound of palms smacking together. Then Marcus continued, "Good. Better anyway. You've got to have a strong handshake but not too strong. A black man around here has to show he's worth a conversation but can't be too dominant, okay? You do that in a handshake but you cannot be the head Negro in charge around these people. Or at least that's kind of what my business teacher said." Anthony laughed and replied, "Always gotta tell us somethin' about school, huh? Whatever, common Elijah. I'll show you the best ways to get around the halls without getting stopped. Now what did your fucking teacher tell you about that, Marcus? Was it on the chapter about how to be a black businessman and *not* get arrested?" Their laughter at this last comment faded as their footsteps rescinded down the hall.

When I asked Anthony and Marcus about the inter-action in a follow up interview, they explained that this inter-action of respectability politics was normal "Crew business." and promptly provided another example where they saw a student in the cafeteria who was alone and seemed to need support. This student was white and in a wheelchair. They explained that the Crew functioned to help as many kids as possible, although they admitted that they specifically targeted youth of color. The intentional infrastructure of the Crew toward these ends was surprisingly specific and they were able to articulate in detail the positions of each student in the group, from a lookout to an emissary. Each student's role played to his strengths, whether it was being empathetic to new students' needs or teaching the "right way" of being a male of color in a predominantly White institution, each member of the Crew performed tasks they believed would help marginalized students feel safe, recognized, and included at school.

Although Anthony's remarks about learning how to avoid arrest were made with a degree of sarcasm and humor, Crew members often expressed their frustration with racial profiling on the part of students, staff and administration not only as a hindrance to their academic lives but in their ability to enact tasks as Crew members intended to create a more inclusive school environment. This was significant for two reasons. The first speaks to a question of which spaces students could use to resist sociocultural norms and values in the school. Derrick noted that, while he understood the need for students to remain in predesignated areas during the school day, there were no areas allocated for students of color to teach others how to socialize in white spaces. Although they were aware that their sociocultural context implicitly and explicitly taught students of color how to "be" in school, they also recognized that places of open resistance to the school-taught, self-fulfilling prophecies around ways of being and knowing in school for students of color were absent. They could work to help other students of color negotiate marginalizing Anglo schooling but did not have a place to openly resist such structures or practices.

Second, one of the advertised pillars of school culture at the time of the study was "Every student, Every time," an understanding meant to convey that faculty, staff, and administration recognized and actively worked to reinforce the notion that every student throughout the school was valued in every inter-action. The Crew, however, noted that their approach to this moto, socializing their fellow students of color school patterns and policies, was often labeled as "bad behavior." This is predominantly due to how place was constructed in this school, an understanding that mirrors the construction of space and place in many institutional geographies (e.g., Foley, 1990; Goffman, 1961; Nespor, 1997). The Crew had identified the corridors of the school as the primary and safest location for conducting Crew business and meetings, a place where students in general, and students of color in specific, were expressly not to congregate.

The label of "bad behavior" was significant for Crew members because most members were already on the school's "discipline ladder" for actions that administration perceived as not following school conduct. This behavior included the Crew's consistent presence in the hallways for, as administrators explained, "being wanderers." This behavior was understood as a possible security issue by administrators while it was viewed as a necessity by Crew members for conducting Crew business. This is not to say that students' decision to be present in the halls was not at once a possible security issue while being a necessity for Crew work. It should also be noted that such movement in the halls was not always an expression of Crew work but, rather, an opportunity for students to be away from class. As Nespor (1997) notes, the knot of schooling gives way to all these possibilities as factors that tie up the social relationships in schools. Further, as explored through scholarship on the school-to-prison pipeline (Christle, Jolivette, & Nelson, 2005), Crew members articulated frustration with the tension between knowing that smaller offenses were more likely to place them further on the discipline ladder while wanting to be a part of grassroots change in the building for students of color.

Their efforts were therefore largely unknown by staff and administration at best and, at worst, Crew members felt as though these efforts only precipitated more punishment. As students struggled with their value in the larger scope of the school, rather than being understood as working to help peers better negotiate the school—something administrators ironically often noted they had more help in conveying to students of color—the punishment they received for Crew business cast an impression of an absence of care from the systems of schooling on their attempts to attend to injustices in the school.

"Bus Your Tray, Boy!": Living With and Against a Tide of Racism and Sensuous Curriculum

Wozolek: So it sounds to me like you're also talking about unequal treatment that's going on as well?

James: Yeah

Wozolek: Darius, how does that kind of stuff make you feel?

Darius: It makes me mad a little bit. Cuz I remember freshman year. We were sitting in lunch and, the table behind me, the kid got up to throw his tray away and he tossed it at the garbage can and it completely missed. And it made a huge mess. Then then, like, I saw him do it and I didn't pay any attention to it and I kept eating and a principal walked up to my table, pointed at me...urgh! Specifically, and told me to pick it up. I just looked at him like, "Why am I picking up some other kid's mess?" and I told the principal who did it. I pointed to the kid and everything and was like, "That kid did it." He was like, "Well.. I want you to pick it up, boy." I was like, "No! I'm not going to pick up some other kid's trash." He's like, "So, all right, so you're being insubordinate? Go to the office." I was like, "Ok." And then I ended up with getting two after school detentions for defying an administrator or somethin' like that.

In group interviews, James and Darius often expressed their frustration with being considered "less than slaves" as biracial students. They noted that their place in the formal curricula they learned, knowledge in texts and assessments for example, was as absent as the places in the school designed for the kind of social justice they were enacting through their work as Crew members. James, for example, argued that, in his experiences, African Americans were either studied "in chains or breaking them" in school. Additionally, he often expressed that even this limited inquiry into African American contributions to United States history classes left out biracial histories. In complete exasperation, James argued that because biracial people were considered the "bastard children of rape that history and teachers want to forget that [they] are the unspoken joke of society" and that this made it "okay for people to treat [biracial students] like shit because ... you're less than a nigger but you'll never be a cracker." This lack of curricular engagement with African American narratives in general and biracial histories in particular resonated negatively among the Crew. They wanted to find their value in the formal curriculum but instead found a space of curricular absence that promoted feelings of "neither/nor" for biracial ways of being and knowing. By this I mean that their Anglo roots were devalued by their African American histories and the curriculum negated the value of their narratives of color. They were neither White enough to be valued in the curriculum nor Black enough to be recognized as a significant part of historical understandings.

The Crew were clear in their articulation of the multiple ways that these absences affected their ways of being and knowing. Such arguments are closely aligned with DuBois' (1926) critique centered on aesthetics and race, Bethune (1938) and Lorde's dialogues focused on Black knowledges, and other seminal texts that argue for the inclusion, and the detrimental consequences, of absent Black histories in the American curriculum (e.g., Cooper, 1892; Gordon, 1993; Watkins, 2001; Woodson, 1933). Foundational scholars in the African American intellectual tradition (Cooper, 1892; DuBois, 1926; Woodson, 1933) often employed metaphors that describe the suffocation of African American students that ultimately end in their ontological and epistemological death to enunciate the negative impact of White, male-dominated curricula in school. This impact does not exist in a historical vacuum, nor did this curriculum exist as a monolithic structure in schooling. There are several players between the system itself and the local actors that engender and maintain the local and less local impact of the curricula in school. Racism-as-affect in this case existed between the bodies of the students and the body of the curriculum. The "sucker punch of privilege" in this case was dealt by the curriculum and those who delivered (teachers) and sanctioned (administrators) curricular ideas and ideals.

An understanding that curriculum affects students is certainly not new (e.g., Cooper, 1892; hooks, 1994; Jackson, 1968; Windfield, 2007; Woodson, 1933). Additionally, contemporary scholarship has expanded the multiple ways that curriculum can affect students, with an understanding that curriculum is inter-active (Gershon, 2013b; Schwab, 1969; Springgay & Freedman, 2012). By this I mean that the curricula (formal, hidden, null, enacted, delivered) is in constant inter-action with students, staff, administration, parents, historical, and contemporary contexts. Sensuous curriculum, how students learn through the sensorium of classrooms in ways that are rooted in the nexus of sociocultural and deeply personal histories (Gershon, 2011), is played out through racialized ideas and ideals for the Crew in the everydayness of schooling. This was significant not only for members of the Crew and other marginalized groups in the building who learned through multiple forms of the sensorium about the school's perceived value of their ways of being and knowing. Additionally, it also impacted Anglo students and staff. In other words, these lessons of sociocultural norms and values impact Anglo understandings of being and normalize hegemonic ideas and ideals. Darius' narrative that focused on the cafeteria is but one example of how staff negatively acknowledged and viewed the presence of students of color in the school and used their power to reinforce these understandings for both the students of color and the Anglo students who observed the situation.

The null curriculum (Eisner, 1985) is generally discussed in terms of what is absent, or what is not taught in schools. The Crew, for example, was generally concerned with the lack of absences of African American voices in the curriculum and, in specific, about the dearth of biracial perspectives in school. As argued in curriculum studies, the null curriculum often functions as an erasure for marginalized voices (Flinders, Noddings & Thornton, 1986; Kridel, 2010; Pinar, 1995). Students were impacted by the null curriculum as it, and those complicit in teaching it, consistently erased and delegitimized the presence of voices of color in schools. Although the null curriculum is not taught, its presence is always active in the ways it shapes the ways of being and knowing for students and staff. In this case, the absence of biracial narratives in the curriculum served as an active marker for the significance of these students in the school and broader community. The Crew was therefore a sociocultural marker of the null curriculum in metaphoric and literal ways. The physical removal of students of color from school, as discussed in terms of detentions, suspensions and, ultimately, the school-to-prison pipeline (Christle, Jolivetten & Nelson, 2005), are some of the multiple ways that the removal of this marker for the null curriculum is carried out daily. The students who participated in the Crew became living examples of the null curriculum in this case. They were not formally recognized and, therefore, were often removed and no longer a part of the acknowledged narrative in schooling.

As heard in the second file in this chapter, students noted their presence as "doom" at school. This sense of literally being (enacting) doom can be thought of as the school's difficulty completely removing students whose presence visually represented the absence of a null curriculum. Though the null curriculum is often discussed in passive terms, in other words, what is not taught and therefore impacts students and staff, here I am attending to the ways that the curriculum is also in-action. Racism-as-affect is therefore the multiple, aggressive ways that the null curriculum landed on the bodies of marginalized students and was expressed by their presence regardless of either their desire or awareness. From this perspective, a sensuous curriculum of racialized ideas and ideals, or the ways that students learned through what they felt, can be attributed to the null curriculum landing on the bodies of the children who represented that-which-cannot-be-taught lessons in school.

CONCLUSION: AVOIDING THE HIT

It's weird. If I tell you I didn't do it, why bring me in three days in a row to basically try and tell me that I did do it when I know I didn't do it and it's not a big deal. But something that is a big deal, kids just have to write a letter and they are off the hook.

File can be heard at: bit.ly/half-breeds4

The war of the half-breeds as enacted through the Crew's battle for social justice in their school was a way for biracial students to intellectually cope with the daily aggressions they experienced. It was also a way to actively push back at the sensuous curriculum of racism-as-affect that constantly and consistently hit students in school. For the Crew, an awareness of the multiple, fluid ways that curriculum interacted with their ways of being and knowing was significant because it meant they could find paths of resistance against or ways to move around being metaphorically. Or, as heard in the last file above, the ways they were physically hit by privilege. Anglo students and staff that had the privilege to ignore how students of color in general, and biracial students in specific, were similarly impacted by racism-as-affect but in the positive: they maintained racisms because it took so little effort to gain so much. In so doing, where Anglo students enacted what DuBois (1926) called the "distorted ugliness" (p. 9) of schooling, students of color were hit by the ugliness of racism.

While schools use the null curriculum to erase narratives of what those in power consider to be sociocultural ugliness, students like those in the Crew have no choice but to continue embodying the physical representation of null curricula, a presence that is further marginalized because it makes explicit that which those in power have worked hard to avoid, racist and racialized formal curriculum for example. Studying sensuous curriculum therefore stands as a reminder of how curriculum in action falls on marginalized bodies and being. As racialized violence continues to fall on bodies of color in and outside of schools, recognizing how racism-as-affect lands ontologically on all participants in school becomes all the more significant. From Woodson's (1933) warning of how educational lynching in schools normalizes physical lynching outside of schools, narratives like those of the Crew underscore how sensuous curricula of racism ontologically suffocates students of color. From this perspective, attention to sensuous curricula can be deeply valuable in their ability to serve as strong indicators of how we continue to normalize the sucker punch of privilege and violence it engenders across contexts every day.

REFERENCES

Agar, M. H. (1996). *The professional stranger: An informal introduction to ethnography* (2nd ed.). San Diego, CA: Academic Press.

Ahmed, S. (2010). Happy objects. In M. Gregg & G. J. Seigworth (Eds.), *The affect theory reader* (pp. 29–51). Durham, NC: Duke University Press.

Baldwin, J. (1962). *The fire next time.* New York, NY: The Dial Press.

Behar, R. (1996). *The vulnerable observer: Anthropology that breaks your heart*. Boston, MA: Beacon Press.

Bethune, M. M. (1938). Clarifying our vision with the facts. *Journal of Negro History, 7*(2), 10–15.

Bethune, M.M. (1939). What does American democracy mean to me? In K. Ellis & S. Smith (Eds.), *Say it plain: Live recordings of the 20th century's great African-American speeches.* Retrieved February 16, 2017, from http://americanradioworks.publicradio.org/features/sayitplain/transcript.html

Christle, C. A., Jolivette, K., & Nelson, C. M. (2005). Breaking the school to prison pipeline: Identifying school risk and protective factors for youth delinquency. *Exceptionality: A Special Education Journal, 13*(2), 69–88.

Cooper, A. J. (1892). *A voice from the south (by a black woman from the south).* Xenia: OH: Aldine Printing House.

DuBois, W.E.B. (1903). *The souls of black folk.* Chicago, IL: McClurgand Co.

DuBois, W.E.B. (1926). Criteria of Negro art. *The Crisis, 32,* 290–297.

Eisner, E. (1985). The educational imagination: On the design and evaluation of school programs (2nd ed.). New York, NY: Macmillan.

Foley, D. E. (1990). *Learning capitalist culture: Deep in the hearts of the Tejas.* Philadelphia, PA: University of Pennsylvania Press.

Flinders, D. J., Noddings, N., & Thornton, S. J. (1986). The null curriculum: Its theoretical basis and practical implications. *Curriculum Inquiry, 16*(1), 33–42.

Geertz, C. (1973). *The interpretation of cultures.* New York, NY: Basic.

Gershon, W. S. (2009). *The collaborative turn: Working together in qualitative research.* Rotterdam: Sense.

Gershon, W. S. (Ed.). (2011). Sensual curriculum: Understanding curriculum of and through the senses. [Special Issue] *Journal of Curriculum Theorizing, 27*(2).

Gershon, W. S. (2013a). Sonic cartography: Mapping, space, place, race and identity in an urban middle school. *Taboo: The Journal of Culture and Education, 13*(1), 21–45.

Gershon, W. S. (2013b). Resonance, affect, and ways of being: Implications of sensual curriculum for educational theory and urban first graders' literacy practices. *The Journal of School and Society*.

Gershon, W. S. (2013c). Vibrational affect: Sound theory and practice in qualitative research. *Cultural Studies? Critical Methodologies, 13*(4), 257–262.

Goffman, E. (1961). *Asylums: Essays on the social situation of mental patients and other inmates.* New York, NY: Doubleday.

Gordon, B. (1993). African-American cultural knowledge and liberatory education: Dilemmas, problems, and potentials in a postmodern American society. *Urban Education, 27*(4), 448–470.

Harvey, D. (1973). *Social justice and the city: Geographies of justice and social transformation*. Athens, GA: The University of Georgia Press.

Heath, S. B. (1983). *Ways with words: Language, life, and work in communities and classrooms.* Cambridge, England: The University of Cambridge Press.

hooks, b. (1994). *Teaching to transgress: Education as the practice of freedom*. New York, NY: Routledge.

Jackson, P. W. (1968). *Life in classrooms.* New York. NY: Holt, Rinehart & Winston.

Kridel, C. (Ed.). (2010). *Encyclopedia of curriculum studies* (Vol. 1). Thousand Oakes, CA: SAGE.

Lorde, A. (1984). *Outsider sister: Essays & speeches by Audre Lorde.* Berkeley, CA: Crossing Press.

Massey, D. (2005). *For space*. London, England: SAGE.

Metz, M. H. (1978). *Classrooms and corridors: The crisis of authority in desegregated secondary schools.* Los Angeles, CA: University of California Press.

Mitchell, R. W., Fasching-Varner, K. J., Albert, K. A. & Allen, C. M. (Eds.). (2014). *Racial battle fatigue in higher education: Exposing the myth of post-racial America.* Landham, MD: Rowman & Littlefield.

Nespor, J. (1997). *Tangled up in school: Politics, space, bodies, and signs in the educational process.* Mahwah, NJ: Erlbaum.

Page, R. (1991). *Lower-track classrooms: A curricular and cultural perspective.* New York, NY: Teachers College Press.

Pinar, W. F. (1995). *Understanding curriculum: An introduction to the study of historical and contemporary curriculum discourses* (Vol. 17). New York, NY: Peter Lang.

Powell, K. (2010). Making sense of place: Mapping as multisensory research method. *Qualitative Inquiry, 16*(7), 539–555.

Rist, R. (1973). *The urban school: A factory for failure.* Cambridge, MA: MIT Press.

Schwab, J. J. (1969). The practical: A language for curriculum. *The School Review, 78*(1), 1–24.

Smith, W. A., Yosso, T. J., & Solórzano, D. G., (2006). Challenging racial battle fatigue on historically white campuses: A critical race examination of race-related stress. In C. A. Stanley (Ed.), *Faculty of color teaching in predominantly white colleges and universities* (pp. 299–327). Bolton, MA: Anker.

Soja, E. W. (2010). *Seeking spatial justice*. Minneapolis, MN: University of Minnesota Press.

Springgay, S., & Freedman, D. (2012). *Mothering a bodied curriculum: Emplacement, desire, affect.* Toronto, ON: University of Toronto Press.

Stewart, K. (2007). *Ordinary affects.* Durham, NC: Duke University Press.

Stoller, P. (1997). *Sensuous scholarship.* Philadelphia, PA: University of Pennsylvania Press.

Tatum, B. D. (2003). "*Why are all the Black kids sitting together in the cafeteria?": And other conversations about race.* New York, NY: Basic Books.

Watkins, W. H. (2001). *The white architects of black education: Ideology and power in America 1865–1954.* New York, NY: Teachers College Press.

Willis, P. (1977). *Learning to labor: How working class kids get working class jobs*. New York, NY: Columbia University Press.

Winfield, A. G. (2007). *Eugenics and education in America: Institutionalized racism and the implication of history, ideology, and memory.* New York, NY: Peter Lang.

Wozolek, B. (2014). What are you anyway? Racial fatigue as daily experience in public schools. In R. W. Mitchell, K. J. Fasching-Varner, K. A. Albert, & C. M. Allen (Eds.), *Racial battle fatigue in higher education: Exposing the myth of post-racial America* (pp. 17–20). Lanham, MD: Rowman & Littlefield.

Wozolek, B., Varndell, R., & Speer, T. (2015). Are we not fatigued?: Queer battle fatigue at the intersection of heteronormative culture, *International Journal of Curriculum and Social Justice, 1*(1), 186–214.

Woodson, C. G. (1933). *The mis-education of the Negro.* Retrieved from https://historyisaweapon.com/defcon1/misedne.html

CHAPTER 5

BLACKNESS, LOVE, AND SENSUOUSNESS AS PRAXIS

Valerie Kinloch and Carlotta Penn
University of Pittsburgh

"To be sensual, I think, is to respect and rejoice in the force of life."
(Baldwin, 1962, p. 43).

"I am a stranger/learning to worship the strangers/around me."
(Jordan, 2005, p. 3).

According to writer and social critic James Baldwin (1962), "to be sensual"—that is, the act, disposition, practice, and stance of being sensuous, loving, conscious, and committed to human life and varied human experiences—reflects an obligation to being present in every aspect of the world. He explains, "the word sensual is not intended to bring to mind quivering dusky maidens or priapic black studs" (pp. 42–43). Instead, the word is a reference "to something much simpler and much less fanciful. To be sensual, I believe, is to respect and rejoice in the force of life, of life itself, and to be *present* in all that one does, from the effort of loving to the making of bread" (p. 43). Being sensual, then, requires that people learn to "respect" life just as much as we learn to "rejoice" in it, that we are

Sensuous Curriculum:
Politics and the Senses in Education, pp. 85–98

purposeful and caring, that we live with intention, and that we love with presence. Yet we are aware that the use of the term, sensual, can never (and should not) erase or make invisible its larger connection and devastating history with respect to racist, sexist, and misogynist behaviors that are rightly attached to it. For the sexualization of girls and women as well as the historical and current-day othering of disenfranchised people in this country alone require humanizing languages and discourses that attend to power, politics, safety, justice, and civil rights. Thus, we understand Baldwin's use of the term "sensual" as a powerful action-oriented concept that rejects sexualization (e.g., priapic Black studs) and that parallels to sensuousness (e.g., respecting, rejoicing, living, loving).

The concept, *sensuous* (as opposed to sensual), and our employment of it are intended to evoke and provoke a stimulation of the senses that support varied ways of being, doing, knowing, and acting in the world. So, too, are they intended to embody and describe actions and behaviors that reflect an unwavering commitment to human life, human living, and human loving. In other words, to be sensuous is to learn to live with, love, and "worship the strangers/around me/whoever you are/whoever I may become" (p. 3), as poet, essayist, and activist June Jordan (2005) explains, *through* the effort of loving and *with* an awareness of who we are in relation to who others are in the world. In this way, we learn to deeply listen to, care about, stand alongside, and forge coalitions with others in the pursuit of justice and in the ongoing process of being and becoming more fully human. This type of sensuousness moves us toward becoming more whole in the doing, knowing, living, and loving of life. It also encourages us to willingly and courageously seek ways to better understand the significance of loving ourselves as we also come to love others who we once may have viewed as "strangers" (Jordan, 2005, p. 3). In other words, sensuousness must be directed by love and calls for justice, particularly for Black and other disenfranchised people in a world that seeks to maintain a tenacious grip on our freedom.

What, then, does it mean to be/become sensuous, especially in the presence of strangers? What are some of the ways Black people in the United States practice and embody sensuousness under hostile, dangerous, and even deadly conditions? How can Black people "rejoice in the force of life, of life itself" (Baldwin, 1962, p. 43) within public spaces that regularly refuse to affirm the validity, value, and sacredness of our very own lives and cultural, educational, intellectual, and sociopolitical histories? To ask it another way, is there any promise of the sensuous, or of sensuousness, as educational praxis for Black people? These questions guide the very purpose of this chapter and frame our approach to understanding sensuousness as connected to Blackness, love, and praxis.

More specifically, in this chapter we consider meanings of sensuousness by drawing on the scholarship and/or lives of James Baldwin, Mary McLeod Bethune, Angela Davis, Martin Luther King, Jr., bell hooks, June Jordan, and, among other Black activists and scholars, Audre Lorde. Their activism, community engagements, and scholarly contributions to education call for a disruption of faulty and racist standards of normalization that overtly advantage discourses of whiteness (e.g., monolingualism, monoculturalism, privilege, unequal distributions of power, static readings of identity) and that explicitly disadvantage discourses of Blackness (e.g., Black identities, cultural practices, intellectual traditions, linguistic ways of being, Black love). It is this disruption that we examine by insisting on the important role sensuousness plays in revolutionizing how Black people "act on what they know" (Baldwin, 1962, p. 9) by directing our gaze onto Blackness and love. To begin, we focus on freedom and sensuousness.

BLACK FREEDOM, BLACK SENSUOUSNESS

Countless people in the United States and across the world have organized, waged protests, fought, and died for Black people's freedom. Manifestos, meditations, community-generated pamphlets, newspapers, poetry collections, open letters, works of fiction and nonfiction, and other published and unpublished texts calling for Black people's freedom fill the still growing canon of writings on Black life. For example, in "I Dream a World," Langston Hughes (1941/1994) shared his dream for a world "where all/will know sweet freedom's way" and where "every man is free" (p. 311). Nikki Giovanni (2003), in her poem titled, "Revolutionary Dreams," initially imagined a world in which freedom would result from her "taking over america to show/these white folks/how it should be done," but she came to recognize her "dreams of being a natural woman" could, in fact, ignite "a revolution" (p. 106). It is a sentiment that echoes what Zora Neale Hurston (1937/1990) in her novel *Their Eyes Were Watching God* described as a type of freedom that arose at sundown when Black people, who "had been tongueless, earless, eyeless conveniences all day long" could now "hear things and talk" (p. 1) as they "passed nations through their mouths" (p. 2).

In his famous "I Have a Dream" speech, Martin Luther King, Jr. (1963) insisted that freedom required an indictment of the United States government because its "manacles of segregation and the chains of discrimination" relegated Black people to "exile in his own land" (p. 217). And, still, Black people are not free and have not reached the Promise Land, as Ta-Nehisi Coates (2015) describes in *Between the World and Me*. The mythological dream—whether for freedom, equality, or access—has not materialized for Black people because the dream "rests on our backs, the bedding made from our bodies" (p. 11). In fact, the dream, in Coates' analysis, seeks to squelch and destroy the hopes of Black life because despite the imminent, deadly threats to our bodies, the reality is "that this is your country, that this is your world, and that this is your body, and you must find some way to live within all of it" (pp. 11–12).

Collectively, these writings on and about freedom, among so many others, bring to the fore the perpetual struggle of Black people to acquire and maintain civil and human rights in a country that daily attacks Black bodies, seeks to render invisible Black lives, and unapologetically assaults Black love. Sensuousness—the use of all of our senses to breath life into otherwise unbearable situations, the capacity to engage in sense-making in connection with lived experiences, and the ability to love as a conscious, purposeful, and transformative act—becomes ever so important in cultivating, maintaining, and sustaining Black life and Black (self and collective) love.

These writings also push us to consider the value, role, and use-ability of centering sensuousness in discussions about, writings on, movements toward, and fights for freedom by and for Black people. While centering sensuousness, particularly in discussions of teaching, learning, research, and curriculum, places attention on the senses, on sense-making, and on experiential ways of knowing, it is equally important that sensuousness is situated within a larger realm. This realm needs to attend to critical perspectives, to research as multi-sensorial, to the personal and/as the political, to love, and to connections among art, politics, human suffering, human life, and lived experiences, a realm of what is and what might be (Baldwin, 1962; DuBois, 1926; Davis, 1983; James, 1998; Jordan, 2005; Pink, 2015; Stovall, 2006).

It is in these and other such ways that June Jordan's (2005) decision to "worship the strangers/around me" (p. 3) connects to James Baldwin's (1962) choice to "respect and rejoice in the force of life … to be *present* in all that one does" (p. 43), just as much as it gestures to Langston Hughes' (1941/1994) desire to "know sweet freedom's way" (p. 311). Such interconnected choices and conscious movements, then, reflect an engagement with and in the world that, for ethnographer Sarah Pink (2015), "accounts for how sensory ways of experiencing and knowing are integral both to the lives of people" and to the ways of conducting research from multi-sensorial perspectives (p. xi).

Although this might be debatable—given that there are, possibly, multiple and conflicting perspectives on what Black love and sensuousness are and what they embody—we strongly contend that Jordan, Baldwin, and Hughes did not rely on the sensuous to speak of freedom in the abstract. Instead, they relied on the sensuous to move toward freedom in ways that reject "erasure of racialized public memory; that is, race reified and universalized becomes transparent, invisible and normalized" (Young & Braziel, 2007, p. 5). Their respective writings and the ways they lived their lives emphasize the visibility of race and racial memory as well as the hope for freedom and for life, which are connected to our varied ways and processes of being, knowing, and doing (e.g., for/with self, for/with others). Thus, the power of the sensuous is to evoke feelings that spark critical action and necessary reaction, and that provoke social change in spaces that are hostile to, and dangerous for, Black people. This is the case for Black people in the United States, particularly, and throughout the world, generally. Hence, the significance of social justice movements such as Black Lives Matter in protecting, respecting, honoring, and loving Black lives and rejecting all forms of Black hate (see also other contemporary justice movements and concerns that center Black and Brown lives, including #FlintWaterCrisis, #NoDAPL, Occupy Movement, Chicago Teachers' Strike, and the increasing amounts of dangerous anti-Indigenous policies, practices, and interactions). The power of the sensuous and sensuousness is to love, to resist, and to act courageously and bravely for the permanent occupation of human freedom. As an example of engagement with sensuousness, we briefly turn to the imprisonment of Angela Davis and to the open letter written to Davis by James Baldwin.

An Example of Engaging Sensuous Solidarity

On the October 26, 1970 edition of *Newsweek* magazine, Angela Yvonne Davis, a professor, activist, communist, and Black freedom fighter with close ties to the Black Panther Party and a track record of resistance to state-sanctioned oppression, was pictured on the magazine's cover, in chains. Such an image of Davis, for some people, evoked feelings of threat, violence, and criminality. From being featured in *Newsweek* magazine to being written about in *The Chicago Tribune, The Los Angeles Times, The New York Times, Reader's Digest,* and *Time* magazine, Davis did become a symbol of revolutionary violence and danger for some people. For many others, however, she became an important physical representation of Black Power and civil rights in this country and around the world.

When her picture appeared on the cover of *Newsweek,* she was in prison awaiting trial on kidnapping and murder charges in connection with the death of a judge in California. Although an all-white jury did not convict Davis of the charges, news of her imprisonment led to the formation of an international movement for justice that campaigned to "Free Angela and All Political Prisoners." Of similar significance, in a powerful "Open Letter" written to Davis in November 1970, James Baldwin insisted that the

Newsweek cover was a clear indication that the majority of white America had come to "glory in its chains" rather than find them intolerable (p. 13).

Baldwin's (1970) letter was an explicit call for attention to the fact that there were many people thinking, talking about, and fighting against the imprisonment of Davis, an understanding that also recognized that Davis's fate was undeniably intertwined with his own as well as with those of all oppressed people. Because silence is always "suicidal" for Black people, Baldwin decided to "make as much noise as I can" (p. 14) so that the world would know of the injustice inflicted upon (and being resisted by) Davis and, by extension, Black communities. Although Baldwin professed to loving all people, he recognized that Black people were not considered worthy of love by majority white America. It was for this reason that Baldwin emphasized the presence and importance of Black love, especially in the face of hate, oppression, and violence: "We *do* feel ourselves sufficiently worthwhile to contend even with inexorable forces in order to change our fate ... and the condition of the world!" (p. 18 [original emphasis]).

This calling to love, however, was not one merely of feelings and emotions; it was not *sensual*, as we describe in the opening of this chapter. For this love required wholesale investment of the self in the collective fight for Black people's freedom, a fight that had (and continues to have) widespread implications for the necessity to change the world for all people. Thus, this calling to love was, and remains, *sensuous* in its commitment to being deeply connected to/with other people, to igniting action and demanding justice, and to making racism and racial oppression visible so that it might be more fully and clearly combatted.

Baldwin (1970) concludes his letter by insisting, "We must fight for your life as though it were our own—which it is—and render impassable with our bodies the corridor to the gas chamber. For, if they take you in the morning, they will be coming for us that night" (p. 18). Here, he offers his own body in sacrifice to save Davis' life, for Baldwin is aware that "the enormous revolution in black consciousness ... means the beginning or the end of America" (p. 17), for, if "we know, and do nothing, we are worse than the murderers hired in our name" (p. 18). This commitment on the part of Baldwin and other Black people, a commitment that requires the presence of our full selves (e.g., physically, intellectually, emotionally, spiritually) in the dangerous, tiring battle for liberty, represents quintessential, sacrificial Black love. This represents a form of sensuousness that is concerned with "understanding the human condition" (Gershon, 2011, p. 8) and changing it for the better.

For us, Baldwin's letter to Davis is an artifact of love and a representation of Black sensuousness. To read it is to feel, smell, taste, see, and hear the political climate then in juxtaposition with what it is now, which, unfortunately, feels all too familiar. To read the letter is to also understand how sensuousness inextricably connects to (a) political and personal expressions and (b) acts of solidarity and support, both on and off the battlefield of struggle (e.g., emotionally, figuratively, physically, politically, etc.). This is particularly the case within a majority white society in which many Black people daily encounter violence, racism, and social inequalities, and in which some white people are "still trapped in a history which they do not understand" (Baldwin, 1962/1993, pp. 8–9). It is a point that surfaces throughout Baldwin's (1962/1993) essay, "My Dungeon Shook: Letter to my Nephew on the One Hundredth Anniversary of the Emancipation," in which he writes about a history that has allowed white people to believe in Black inferiority and white superiority, even when "many of them, indeed, know better" (p. 9). Yet, as Baldwin explains, "people find it very difficult to act on what they know. To act is to be committed, and to be committed is to be in danger. In this case, the danger, in the minds of most white Americans, is the loss of identity" (p. 9).

Emphatically, throughout both this essay and his book, *The Fire Next Time*, Baldwin encouraged his nephew, as he urged Angela Davis and his readers, to not become "an immovable pillar" in the quest to help "make America what America must become" (p. 9). He also insisted that people of conscious minds should not be afraid to be guided by the type of love that requires white people "to see themselves as they are, to cease fleeing from reality and begin to change it" (p. 10). This is, in our belief, a deliberate move toward a politicized form of sensuousness that is grounded in freedom, justice, liberty, and love.

One can feel and taste this sensuousness just as much as one can see and hear it, smelling it with and through each inhale of the breath. This sensuousness helps us to make sense of our particular realities at what Gershon (2011) describes as "a fluid intersection of sociocultural norms and values, agency, identity, physiology, awareness, and personal taste" (p. 1). Understanding sensuousness is an attempt to understand, if at all possible, the complexities and nuances of human encounters. It is an outright effort to have, possess, and always sustain one's freedom, in part by understanding that our lives and fates are connected, for better or for worse. Therefore, we are all better off when we are united in a "beloved community" (King, 1957, p. 12) of what we refer to as *SisterBrotherHood.*

Sensuous SisterBrotherHood

An example of what it means to embody sensuousness presents itself in the life of Mary McLeod Bethune, whose vision for the world was guided by "peace, progress, brotherhood, and love" (1955, p. 61). Bethune, an education leader, social justice activist, and founder of the girls' school that later became Bethune-Cookman University in Daytona Beach, Florida, believed that "love builds. It is positive and helpful ... our aim must be to create a world of fellowship and justice where no man's skin, color or religion, is held against him" (p. 59). This type of love has the potential to "transform the world if it were universally practiced" (p. 59). Bethune dreamed of a world wherein the gates of freedom would be forced open and, similar to what Baldwin (1962/1993) came to argue years later, where Black people would no longer confront "tyranny and oppression and race supremacy" (Bethune, 1944, pp. 21–22) because, in fact, they would be free. She was more than aware that Black and other disenfranchised people in the United States were excluded from the Constitutional guarantee of equal participation in a free society, an understanding that caused her to demand that the government welcome them "into the free realm of democratic citizenship" (p. 24).

Simultaneously, Bethune's (1955) belief in "faith, courage, brotherhood, dignity, ambition, responsibility" (p. 61) pointed to her commitment to securing Black people's freedom. It also represented her attempt to make sense of the world in light of its many contradictions, especially in relation to race, racism, oppression, and justice—an engagement in an active process of sense-making to question and create avenues for Black people's freedom. In so doing, she sought to actively understand the past by, as Sarah Pink (2015) argues, determining ways we can "engage with our present and ... imagine our futures" (p. 3). For us, this speaks to how Bethune lived within a very sensuous moment that embodied an equally sensuous disposition in the fight for justice and Black life.

Such a focus on sense-making, freedom, and love lies at the heart of Dr. Martin Luther King, Jr.'s (1957) philosophy, whose belief that "the only way to ultimately change humanity and make for the society that we all long for is to keep love at the center of our lives" (p. 13). King implored us all to practice agape, or unconditional and sacrificial, love if we truly desire to "move from the bleak and desolate midnight of a man's inhumanity to man to the bright and glittering daybreak of freedom and justice" (p. 15), which is a sensuous love that emphasizes "understanding, creative, redemptive good will for all men" (p. 13). According to King's philosophy, agape love, coupled with nonviolent resistance, has the power to open the hearts and awaken the consciousness of all people such that justice can be realized and actualized. This type of love is powerful, for it has the potential to motivate people to be committed to fighting for justice in a way that "disarms the adversary ... exposes his moral defenses, weakens his morale, and at the same time works on his conscious" (King, 1961, p. 164). As adversaries are disarmed, new pathways for justice—in theory, practice, and praxis—might be revealed, created, and sustained in ways that fully center sensuousness and the sensory experience. Such pathways integrate and affirm multiple knowledge and cultures, and diverse ways of knowing and doing as connected to Black life, Black love, and Black civil rights.

What do these two examples—of Bethune and King—have to do with sensuousness? If the sensuous represents the human experience, and if it is a deliberate stance, act, and practice related to human life and human love, then it inscribes and is inscribed by the fabrics of the everyday. We know what we know, and we become who we become, through sensory information and because of our sensuousness. We fight for justice and engage in acts of love that are revolutionary in the face of oppression, aggression, and attempts at wholesale erasure because our senses and sense-making processes direct us to do so, with, for, and because of others. And we do this work, as King and Bethune so modeled for us, because, we hope, we have a "vision of a world of Peace, Progress, Brotherhood and Love" (Bethune, 1955, p. 61). Sensuousness directs us to engage in the world as a means to change it, and one way to change it is by locating the sensuous within praxis—within our teaching, learning, and curriculum work.

A SENSUOUS PRAXIS

Many Black writers, educators, and activists have emphasized the importance of sensuousness in the realm of education. For example, bell hooks (1994) encourages educators not to submit to the mind/body split in our practice, for the false division of the self is a misguided tradition handed down through generations that makes for a "disembodied spirit" and an incomplete person. In order to be "whole in the classroom, and as a consequence wholehearted" (p. 193), hooks believes we must acknowledge passion in our pedagogy, the erotic and the realities of the physical body. It is a sentiment that resonates with Audre Lorde's (1984) ruminations on the erotic and a dominant ideology of falsely separating the erotic—which Lorde suggests is fundamentally a powerful form of love—from the spiritual and political. In its stead, Lorde contends that a full embrace of the erotic opens us up to the truest path to knowledge, joy, and understanding of ourselves, with ourselves, and with others: "The erotic is the nurturer or nursemaid of all our deepest knowledge" (p. 56).

In her own acknowledgement of the erotic, hooks (1994) suggests that an engagement in educational exchanges that inspire students and teachers alike would help us adjust "our habits of being and ways of living outside the classroom" (p. 194). For, it is with our full selves present, especially our willingness to give and receive love, that hooks believes critical thinking, joy, and meaningful relationships will thrive. In our contemporary educational context, the value of love, passion, and critical reflection in the classroom surface when we demonstrate our deep care for others and for ourselves.

When we more vigilantly invest in life habits and commitments, we move society in the direction of social and racial justice. A classroom, bell hooks insists, should exist as a site of possibility where, "we have the opportunity to labor for freedom, to demand of ourselves and our comrades, an openness of mind and heart that allows us to face reality even as we collectively imagine ways to move beyond boundaries, to transgress" (p. 207).

Another central element of Black sensuousness is the importance of self-love and self-care (van Gelder, Davis, & Davis, 2016; Lorde, 1988). As Audre Lorde (1988) so poignantly writes, "Caring for myself is not self-indulgence, it is self-preservation, and that is an act of political warfare (p. 131). Indeed, by prioritizing self-care, Lorde also suggests we become better able to "extend ourselves to each other and to call upon each other's strengths" (p. 124) in ways that can be life-saving and life-changing. Lorde's words are as powerful today as they were when she first penned them. In fact, after a lifetime of "fighting" for the liberation of oppressed communities, Angela Davis echoes Lorde's appreciation of self-love in the movement for collective freedom. She states, "self-care and healing and attention to the body and the spiritual dimension—all of this is now a part of radical social justice struggles" (as cited in van Gelder, Davis, & Davis, 2016). However, to love and to care for the self are not to ignore, neglect, or take-for-granted the *SisterBrotherHood*. Historically, Black people have never had a choice but to recognize that the system of racial oppression that still operates today—a system that disadvantages and oppresses, demeans and dehumanizes us—connects our fate one to another without regard for the depth, beauty, nuance, and complexity of Blackness. For this reason, Lorde (1997) wrote to activist and author Assata Shakur, "I dream of your freedom/as my victory/and the victory of all dark women/who forego the vanities of silence" (p. 252). In many ways parallel to the words James Baldwin offered to Angela Davis, Audre Lorde's sentiments to Assata Shakur are not merely heartfelt; they are a provocation that suggests a type of sensuous connection one to another without distinguishing one's freedom as inseparable from another. For, this type of sensuousness is of an undying habit and tendency of feelings, that is breathing, that is smelling, that is tasting, and that is hearing of all the realities of an always evolving sensorium beyond (white) Western dualisms and limitations that is Blackness and Black love. This sensuousness is both *of* and *for* the types of justice that lead to liberation for Black people, a sensuality that connects human life and realities to critical praxis.

A SENSUOUS LIBERATION

Undoubtedly, there is much left to learn from the sensuous engagements of James Baldwin, Angela Davis, Mary McLeod Bethune, Martin Luther King,

Jr., bell hooks, Audre Lorde, and thousands upon thousands of other courageous Black freedom fighters. This is especially the case within a society such as our contemporary condition in the United States that exists and is structured on the continuing exploitation and destruction of Black life. The inseparable lives and work of these liberation fighters make holding "fast to dreams" plausible, particularly in light of Langston Hughes' (1995) warning that "when dreams go/life is a barren field/frozen with snow" (p. 32). Alternatively, sensuous engagement on the battlefield that is a white supremacist, patriarchal, racist, sexist, heteronormative United States of America makes liberation possible in the lives of Black people. There is so much to gain from loving ourselves, loving our family members, loving our friends and neighbors, and especially loving our communities and community members, even, or, as we contend, especially, under hostile, dangerous, and deadly circumstances.

Historically, Black freedom fighters recognize the importance of educational spaces as sites for sensuous liberation. Consider the example of the Oakland Community School,[1] founded in 1970 by Black Panther Party members to develop Black children holistically, with a focus on analysis, collaboration, and community engagement. The goal was to have Black children fully and harmoniously "participate and survive" (Black Panther Party, 1971, p. 2) in society. According to the school's brochure, students learned "the basic principles of living and working together" and practiced the proverb, "each one help one, each one teach one" (p. 3). Youth and adults had "mutual love and respect for one another" (p. 3), worked cooperatively, and practiced a version of democracy whereby power and responsibility were distributed equitably amongst all members of the community. Importantly, educators encouraged children to engage the senses as part of their learning experiences—they were guided by the principle that "in order to be able to transform any situation or thing, one must be in contact with it" (p. 5). Therefore, students were able to "study the physical and social phenomena of their community firsthand and test out their theories for making changes through practical activity" (p. 5). This commitment to equity, harmonious living, and interactive, collaborative learning, exemplifies a sensuous educational praxis.

The aforementioned example also demonstrates the significance of educators today considering the sensuous and sensuousness as central to our critical and reflexive praxis and practices. We must have a commitment to be "involved in research [and other educational engagements] that seeks to intervene in the world, to make change and to have 'impact'" (Pink, 2015, p. 189). We must also understand that "such approaches [should be] oriented towards the future, and need in this sense to consider how a sensory approach can enable us to understand this unknown and uncertain domain" (Pink, 2015, p. 189). Relatedly, we must always be aware of how the senses are at play inside learning communities, and we must individually and communally stand behind the necessity of *feeling* and *emotion* for our literal and metaphoric holistic health. This is how we become human; this is how we remain human. This, too, is how we are made whole in our sense of being and in our knowingness in and of the world, leading to our freedom.

If we are to experience a liberation in our lives, and if we want a sensuous liberation in the lives of our students and their families, then sense-making—as intimately connected to care, love, and resistance—must guide our lives and fights for justice, as well as guide our words, engagements, curricula, policies, and the relationships we cultivate with others inside classrooms and throughout the world. We must ask ourselves: What does it mean to love unconditionally, and will unconditional love lead to our liberation? What does a beloved community *feel* like, and is it enough to pursue in the fight for justice? How can we be vocal and bold in solidarity with those around us who are experiencing isolation, discrimination, and exclusion from the very classrooms and communities that purport to nurture them? How can we develop *SisterBrotherHood* with colleagues, students, caregivers, family members, friends, and even with policymakers and policy-enforcers in light of, and because of, the threats against Blackness? What does it mean to seek peace with "strangers," to borrow June Jordan's (2005) term, who may or may not know peace and love?

To engage in sensuousness is to know that freedom must be a universal right for all people, and especially Black people. This knowing means that we must be so drawn into tasting and smelling freedom just as much as we must be so drawn into seeing, feeling, and hearing the sounds of freedom for self and for others. "The everyday ways of knowing, being and experiencing," according to Pink (2015), "are not just related to the past and present, but rather they are part of the ways in which the future is present in our lives as we live them, and as we ongoingly slip over the edge of the present into the immediate future" (p. 193). Additionally, the sensuousness of freedom and justice also means that we come to make "impassable with our bodies" (Baldwin, 1970, p. 18) those people and practices that seek to destroy Black lives. This is a call to action, particularly for teachers, researchers, administrators, students, and community members who are committed to a "pathway to freedom" when it comes to educational praxis for Black people, a praxis that is not possible without engaging the sensuous. A sensuous liberation is at hand, and this liberation is inexorably connected to a sensuous form of love, a sensuous curriculum, and a sensuous praxis.

NOTE

1. The school went through several stages of development, and was known as The Children's House, Samuel L. Napier Intercommunal Youth Institute, and the Oakland Community School.

REFERENCES

Baldwin, J. (1970). An open letter to my sister, Angela Y. Davis. In A. Davis (Ed.), *If they come in the morning: Voices of resistance* (pp. 11–19). New York, NY: Third World Press.

Baldwin, J. (1993). *The fire next time*. New York, NY: Vintage International. (Original work published 1962)

Bethune, M. M. (1944). Certain unalienable rights. In M. M. Bethune, E. M. Smith, & A. T. McCluskey (Eds.), *Mary McLeod Bethune: Building a better world: Essays and selected documents*. Bloomington, IN: Indiana University Press.

Bethune, M. M. (1955). My last will and testament. IIn M. M. Bethune, E. M. Smith, & A. T. McCluskey (Eds.), *Mary McLeod Bethune: Building a better world: Essays and selected documents*. Bloomington, IN: Indiana University Press.

Black Panther Party. (1971, January). *The Samuel L. Napier Intercommunal Youth Institute*. Retrieved from http://freedomarchives.org/Documents/Finder/DOC513_scans/BPP_Nocal/513.BPPNC.sam.napier.intercommunal.youth.institute.jan.1971.pdf

Coates, T. (2015). *Between the world and me*. New York, NY: Spiegel & Grau.

Davis, A. (1983). *Women, race, and class*. New York, NY: Vintage Books.

DuBois, W.E.B. (1926). Criteria of negro art. Retrieved from http://www.webdubois.org/dbCriteriaNArt.html

hooks, b. (1994). *Teaching to transgress: Education as the practice of freedom*. New York, NY: Routledge.

Gershon, W. (2011). Introduction: Toward a sensual curriculum. *Journal of Curriculum Theorizing, 27*(2), 1–16.

Giovanni, N., & Fowler, V. C. (2003). *The collected poetry of Nikki Giovanni, 1968–1998*. New York, NY: William Morrow.

Hughes, L. (1994). I dream a world. In A. Rampersad (Ed.), *The collected poems of Langston Hughes* (p. 311). New York, NY: Vintage Books. (Originally circulated by the Associated Negro Press (*Amsterdam News*, 1941, p. 14)

Hughes, L., Rampersad, A., & Roessel, D. E. (1995). *The collected poems of Langston Hughes*. New York, NY: Vintage Books.

Hurston, Z. N. (1990). *Their eyes were watching God*. New York, NY: Harper & Row. (Original work published 1937)

James, J. (Ed.). (1998). *The Angela Y. Davis reader*. Malden, MA: Blackwell.

Jordan, J. (2005). These poems. In J. H. Levi & S. Miles (Eds.), *Directed by desire: The collected poems of June Jordan* (p. 3). Port Townsend, WA: Cooper Canyon Press.

King, M. L. (1957). The power of nonviolence. In J. M. Washington (Ed.), *A testament of hope: The essential writings and speeches of Martin Luther King Jr.* (pp. 12–15). New York, NY: HarperOne.

King, M. L. (1961). The time for freedom has come. In. J. M. Washington (Ed.), *A testament of hope: The essential writings and speeches of Martin Luther King Jr.* (pp. 160–166). New York, NY: HarperOne.

King, M. L. (1963). I have a dream. In. J.M. Washington (Ed.), *A testament of hope: The essential writings and speeches of Martin Luther King Jr.* (pp. 160–166). New York, NY: HarperOne.

Lorde, A. (1984). Uses of the erotic: The erotic as power. In *Sister outsider: Essays and speeches* (pp. 53–59). New York, NY: Ten Speed Press.

Lorde, A. (1988). *A burst of light: Essays*. Ithaca, NY: Firebrand Books.

Lorde, A. (1997). *The collected poems of Audre Lorde*. New York, NY: W. W. Norton & Company.

Pink, S. (2015). *Doing sensory ethnography* (2nd ed.). Los Angeles, CA: SAGE.

Stovall, D. (2006). We can relate: Hip hop culture, critical pedagogy, and the secondary classroom. *Urban Education, 41*(6), 585–602.

Van Gelder, S., Davis, A., & Davis, F. (2016, February 18). A radical work of healing: Fania and Angela Davis on a new kind of civil rights activism. *Yes! Magazine: Powerful Ideas Practical Actions.* Retrieved from http://www.yesmagazine.org/issues/life-after-oil/the-radical-work-of-healing-fania-and-angela-davis-on-a-new-kind-of-civil-rights-activism-20160218

Young, J. A., & Braziel, J. E. (2007). *Erasing public memory: Race, aesthetics and cultural amnesia in the Americas.* Macon, GA: Mercer University Press.

CHAPTER 6

THE VISCERAL CURRICULUM

Avi Lessing
Independent Scholar

> You know that song 'If a body catch a body comin' through the rye'? I'd like—"
>
> "It's 'If a body meet a body coming through the rye'!" old Phoebe said. "It's a poem. By Robert Burns." "I know it's a poem by Robert Burns."
>
> She was right, though. It is "If a body meet a body coming through the rye." I didn't know it then, though.
>
> "I thought it was 'If a body catch a body,'" I said.
>
> *Holden talking to his sister Phoebe, The Catcher in the Rye* (Salinger, 1951).

MY MOM'S OFFICE

A third of my mom's clients are therapists like her. One couple seeing her for marriage counseling a few years back began a session by saying, "We think you're secretly the cleaning lady." My mom beamed telling the story back to me. It was one of the best compliments she had ever gotten.

Sensuous Curriculum:
Politics and the Senses in Education, pp. 99–114

"How is that a compliment?" I asked.

"They didn't see me in my role: I was a human being who was *there*. In therapy, you have to talk about something. But the real stuff happens on a totally different level."

She was talking about the experience of being with another person, the experience of *meeting* and *being* in the presence of others beyond what feels predetermined and scripted.

"But how do you know what that different level is and when you're there?" I asked my mom. "And how do your clients know."

"They know because they start to understand ..." She trailed off. "It's difficult to explain in words."

And yet it is this sense of *being*, or *being present* that counts most in her work with clients. When clients are discussing their marriage, their deepest desires and problems, it turns out it is incredibly difficult to experience discomforting thoughts and sensations. It is much easier to revert to the stories they have always told themselves, leave the room, check out, argue, defend, go numb, panic or throw up any number of protective stances that prevent them from fully meeting a moment. On the other hand, if you can deal with difficult material and keep noticing what's happening, with guidance of a skilled therapist, then you have a chance for real transformation.

Which is why mom took the cleaning lady line as a compliment. Not only was she doing great work with this couple, but from the outside eye, it seemed almost easy, like almost anyone could do it.

THE CLASSROOM IN THE SCHOOL

There is a parallel to the experience of being in a classroom. While our aims are not exclusively therapeutic, what students partly take from their experience in school is what it *feels like* to be in their environment—classrooms, hallways, locker rooms. It is this undefined and unexplored territory of the encounters between people in different spaces which might matter most in the ways that are difficult to measure; for example, how we engage or tune out, persist or give up, pursues a passion or take a prescribed route.

Unlike therapists, educators do not have a language, let alone a practice, to even conceive of the relevance of presence, or conversely, distraction in one's teaching. How can we describe what *being there* means? What would it look like not to be there?

Sixteen years of No Child Left Behind and Race to the Top have left us in an educational moment that ensures teachers are ever more concerned about skill preparation than something so abstract as one's presence in relation to another person. And yet, the conversation about how we see, hear, interact, and meet one another in the space (or as is so often the case, do not) is absolutely integral to any learning experience.

For instance: I can trace back my love of writing to my freshmen year English teacher, Mr. Allison. Each quarter, he gave us lined composition books, in which we had journal. Mr. Allison would walk around, in a bowtie and jacket, but because of his proximity, the formality of his clothing somehow made him even more familial. His benevolent and patient presence I can still feel almost 30 years later. I remember other things too: who sat next to me (Matt Miller), how the afternoon light always came in sharply 15 minutes into the period, and how Mr. Allison would then lower the blinds slightly and noiselessly. Also his words about writing stick out—how to generate ideas (through discovery), construct sentences (by eliminating unnecessary words), and to check our grammar using our Strunk and White bibles. I cannot separate what I learned from his presence. "You're a good writer, Lessing," he said to me once late in the year. I do not think I was but him saying so made me want to try.

Experiencing that relationship was the best preparation I could have for being in new experiences and staying ready. In his class, the commotion of high school, the sense of being always behind, disheveled, reacting, and underwater, would for a moment, abate and I could feel time expanding, and my senses expanding with it. For me, this was not merely a blip in the day, but a call towards a more enlightened future. I finally felt firmly where I was.

In school, there is little time to consider the past or the future, let alone be present. Every part of the day in school everyone is supposed to be somewhere doing something. "Keep them busy," one colleague told me my first year of teaching. "The busier they are, the less trouble they can get into." But being busy for the sake of busyness is neither satisfying for students in the present nor effective as preparation for college or for any future profession (at least not one we'd want for our own children). How did we arrive at a schooling system in which there is almost no time to pursue anything with time to deliberate? Where one begins one thing and then get immediately interrupted by another. Rousseau's (1762/ 2013) idea of a learning in which we are "losing time" would strike the followers of utilitarianisms as pointless, verging on lunacy. School is a place to work, home is a place to relax.

It is almost taken for granted that school and life are separate. So many of our students go to schools where they sit in desks constructed from the mid-20th century keeping busy, secretly or not-so-secretly bored, waiting for or needing the day to end. It is why we somehow need an educational movement called 21st century education in the 21st century—as if what stands for progressivism now is merely to get out of the past into the present. It is why an outdated model of psychology, behaviorism, still places teachers and students as opposing forces backed by inane pearls of wisdom, like *don't smile until Christmas* and *start hard then relax* and institutionalized ways of starting (bell ringers) and ending classes (exit quizzes) as if young people were packs of wild animals to control rather than children to care for and teach. No wonder students freak out or freeze up when they see us out in the world. Teacher belong in the boxes of their classroom, not in the world.

Those boxes are further artificialized through a tracking system based supposedly on ability, which are of course impacted by many calculable and incalculable aspects of school beyond the scope of this essay. This tracking has the effect of separating bodies bases on test scores, teacher recommendations, grades, in short, the schooling that came before it. Of course, race and class are often either determiners or a result of this segregation.

How students are evaluated is equally alienating. First, we separate then we grade. Most grading systems at least in high school are based on points that a student does or doesn't accumulate over the course of a semester. Invariably, this leads to an educational system where young people are more concerned with their grades than their learning, the result rather than the experience.

We may read many a study about the effectiveness of mindfulness in schools—to make students more aware, more attentive, (or more insidiously) more compliant, but how many classes or schools across America actually start class with mindfulness or offer students a chance to reflect before jumping into content? Even in my senior elective that values mindful practices, it is far more convenient and involves almost no thinking to take our cue from the bell, take only a half breath, and start talking.

There are so many young people who don't succeed (by any measure) in such a system, who don't connect to their subjects or their teachers, and schooling is primarily something to get through and surmount. Like my mom's clients, our students remain closed, fall back on older patterns of distraction that ensure they will not learn from us. Unlike therapists, we punish students who are not engaged through giving them bad grades.

The rat race meanwhile continues unabated. The teacher and students go from bell to bell, teaching and absorbing material, for a test that results in a grade that will determine whether you can go to college *to actually experience life*. The learning that a student carries with them is too often negligible. Most of what they passively receive, they actively dump into the heap of the forgotten and the unlearned, once the grade has been issued.

Lamentably, the student regards the teacher, the classroom, and the school as predictable, deadened, an unreal purgatory where nobody is really where they are, where everybody is just trying to get through the day, the week, the year without too much commotion, in isolation, in cliques, in an intractable hierarchy. Survival is what matters. And a high GPA.

When teachers and students start counting down the school year ("only 48 days until summer") or the school week ("it's almost Friday") or even the school day ("it's already 7th period") we get a sense of how we typically perceive the school experience. It means evasion, escape, tuning out, present only so far as to be counted as present (who could forget in the movie, *Ferris Bueller's Day Off* [Hughes, 1986], the substitute teacher droning on and on, *Bueller, Bueller)* to register a score in the gradebook. Life, real life, we all understand, happens elsewhere.

One day, I ask my own high school students to raise their hands if they have ever had the experience of coming to class and just tuning out their teacher for the entire period. Invariably, most if not all of the students raise their hands. Next I ask them to raise their hands if they have done this on a regular basis with certain classes, or specific teachers, or on certain days. I am surprised how many hands remain up. As an afterthought I ask how many of them *come to school to tune out*. In the presence of all those raised hands I feel firsthand the crisis of education, the rampant disengagement, low grade despair, and sheer onslaught of distraction that coats every experience or non-experience teachers and students have together.

This all I have experienced firsthand at the high school where I teach, which is one of the top ranked schools in the state of Illinois. What about schools that lack plentiful resources and the committed, talented teachers my school employs? Or what if I asked similar questions to students who were not taking my senior elective, but who have been placed in low track classes? What responses would they give? Schools can operate like mini ghettoes, forcing young people into spaces they do not want to go, keeping them from experiencing the untapped resource they desperately need—the kind of positive experiences that explore, excite, and heighten our sense of being. Too often young people thrive in spite of school rather than because it.

If we want to imagine an education that feels relevant to students' lived lives and not just a stepping stone towards living-in-the-future than we must understand the ways in which *being* and *learning* are inextricably connected from the day school beings in kindergarten.

DROPPING MY CHILDREN OFF AT SCHOOL

My oldest child, Raiva, recently began kindergarten. At the Open House, her teacher attempts to explain to parents what our children will experience the rest of the year. I know I am hearing only the outlines of her experience at school but not understanding the thing itself. The parents barrage my daughter's kindergarten teacher with question after question about the curriculum, the requirements, and what to do at home. Some of them are sensible enough, but many of them verge on insanity (an insanity that America's education system has created). Some of the questions revolve around how to position their children so that they can be admitted to the best selective enrollment high schools in 10 years. The kindergarten teacher stands on the side of the room with her arms crossed. She has not gotten past slide one of her carefully prepared PowerPoint. She assures us she is an *academic* kindergarten teacher.

I walk in-between the miniature desks to the other side of the room and sit down on the heater by the windows. It emits a strange buzzing noise. Or is it raining? I want to ask: *what's the vibe in the class?* Or, *tell me a good story about Ravia*. But by this time, I am tuning out, in the same way I imagine my students do when there is too much information about the future and not enough happening in the present. The Q&A drags on and I focus on my daughter's little desk. Beyond home, this is where she spends the majority of her waking life. The 12 minutes are up (time at Open House like during the school day is carefully regulated, chopped up, and dispersed) and we head out to the parking lot. I try to make eye contact with the teacher, some look to convey compassion, but it is clear, she is just happy to have made it through the gauntlet.

The next day, I drop Raiva off at school. She chatters away in the backseat. I notice it is hard to take a deeper breath, unless I remind myself to do it. At times, being with my children or my students feels like there either isn't time or wherewithal to be in sync with time. Things like finishing a conversation, eating, or going to the bathroom become extraneous.

It had been an anxious transition at school for my daughter and she was finally getting comfortable. Or maybe it was an anxious transition for me and I was finally getting comfortable. It is so hard to tell what the *right* kind of struggle is in parenting, teaching, life, that is, when it is helpful to be uncomfortable and when it is better to be comfortable.

I park the car and we walk hand-in-hand across the street mirroring dozens of other parents and their children doing the same. When we hit the school playground, Raiva lets go, and I watch all the bodies zigzag and fly into an indecipherable pattern of bodies. I think how all around the world this before-school scene plays out at almost every moment in time. I think about how far from home school must seem to her. How far it seems to *me*. I see the woman directing traffic and think suddenly about an article my brother in law sent me recently, the gist of which is how we are all pretending to be adults. Remembering that fact comforts me.

The intensity of the moment crescendos when the bell rings, or rather blares, and we are suddenly separated, the children funneled into lines for their separate classrooms. They are surrounded by each other and yet alone in the world with only one's body to accompany them. Of course Raiva's not thinking that—she is holding her place in line, the sinews of her body stretched, leaning forward. I hug and kiss her goodbye in line and I cannot tell if we hold on extra-long because of her or me. Everything feels shaky.

The playground suddenly empties. I cannot help but feel like I am in a French Film: how the anarchy of the children at play suddenly dissipates. The world feels both small and large, but definitely unfathomable. Halfway back from the parking lot, I realize it is not the world that is shaking. It is me. I stick my arms out: my fingers are trembling. Like I have survived a man-made storm. It is unsettling to experience something so normal on such an intense, visceral level. In the car, I don't turn on the radio, like I normally would.

Is it possible that the least talked about aspect of our existence also gets the least consideration? What it is like being somewhere. And especially in school, where we are so tightly connected to other human beings, where the experience of our bodies matter so much, where it is so hard to stay connected, to experience any given moment, is it not it vital to try and understand what all of these feelings and sensations are about? If we are to understand how young people experience school, we must sort through the immediate and physical experience of being in a classroom and in a school.

THE VISCERAL EXPERIENCE

Mr. Moretti was a teacher who talked about physical sensations, even if it was in a somewhat off-kilter way. He and I shared a room my first year of teaching. I was just out of graduate school, filled up with ideas of Erik Erickson and Karl Marx and Luce Irigary. He was a grizzled veteran. "Now look," he told me the first time we met, "In the morning they're hungry. Don't let them eat in the classroom. Wa-atch that they don't stick gum to the bottom of their desks. Afternoon, sun comes in. They get hot. Don't let them touch the fan."

Moretti spoke in such a way that made you think some wrongdoing had just happened or was about to, and that you could be implicated, if you did not watch yourself. I tried not to take it personally. He was seemingly irritated with everyone, but the effect was more curmudgeonly than misanthropic. He seemed on first impression like a cartoon character of one of those past-their-prime teachers who never should have been in the classroom in the first place, someone who makes you think *wow this guy hates kids.*

My English department chair sure hated him. (I knew this because he had always said, "I hate him," after every time I saw them interact). The truth was more complicated. He *was* grouchy and unapproachable. But many students loved him. His gruffness was a cover for something else. He loved teaching and his students surely felt that.

As comedic as his description of what happens in a classroom were—based, as far as I could tell, on temperature and bodily functions—there was also something incisive about his observations. While he used his knowledge mainly to avoid conflict, create boundaries, and keep the students in their place, he was partially right. They were hungry and they were hot.

Before we talk about overhauling and reforming education it seems vitally important to understand from close range what even happens in a classroom and school on a visceral level. Being hungry or stuffed, hot or cold, peaceful or anxious, matters. Sure you can teach bell to bell but that doesn't mean anybody is paying attention, or cares to.

A *visceral curriculum* would consider all of the things a person feels in school. The visceral experience includes one's physical comfort or discomfort, ability to breathe regularly or not, the times where everything goes whacko inside, either because of some external event (a math problem, a bad interaction in the lunchroom) or something more internal (an insecurity, a paranoid thought). It is what happens to our bodies not just our minds.

As teachers, we are not oriented towards noticing, talking about, or thinking carefully through these aspects of being in school. Teachers and students largely keep these things to themselves, at a great cost. We end up valuing the parts of our experience that have already been validated and deemed successful—the ones that dutifully perform the given task and hopefully score well. But what if, as so often is the case in school, we are trying (and so often failing) to learn something new, what if we have just made our 100th mistake of the day, and we are not handling it very well, how then do we respond to our students and them to us? If we cannot be as fascinated with failure, discomfort, and disorientation as we are with success, then we are only valuing what we already, instead of what we do not know, or what we do not know we do not know. Those moments of not knowing often unlock questions that not only help us learn something new, but prepare us for life, where we continually face the unknowns, even embrace them.

Learning and living are no more separate than cognition and feeling. The mind and the body are not separate entities. They are parts of a larger whole. A visceral experience is the connective tissue between them. It is a potential bridge to splits that were false to begin with.

THE INTELLECTUAL IS NOT SEPARATE FROM THE EMOTIONAL

In Bill Schubert's Curriculum Studies graduate seminar at the University of Illinois, we were going around the room talking about *what we were interested in writing about* for our dissertations. I noticed something in my eye. And then—have you ever had this happen—where you cannot tell if something physically awful is happening which requires you to excuse yourself or if something emotionally terrible is happening in which case it is too embarrassing to excuse yourself? I was somewhere in between those two realities: part of me thought I was about to have a stroke and another part thought I was having a panic attack. If it *was* a panic attack, I thought, might I panic-myself-to-death in a moment of sheer terror which would later be misdiagnosed as stroke?

I sat there dumbstruck in a kind of low-grade, paranoid catatonia pretending that *nothing was happening*.

Some time passed.

I began to think maybe I just had something in my eye after all. I was not dying ("not yet!"). When I thought I probably was not going to die was when I began enjoying the experience. As if thinking I was going to die, not dying, was giving me the feeling of having a second chance at life without the trauma of almost dying. The fear was transforming into just enough discomfort to keep both mundanity and fear on their respective sidelines. Plus, my perceptions were slightly altered. People seemed slightly blurry and in their blurriness paradoxically more clear. The perfect mixture of comfort (I am not going to die) and discomfort (I am experiencing something completely different) turned out to be fascinating. I took a couple of deeper breathes. Everybody and everything was suddenly boundless. Somehow, the fact that this happening in my graduate school class made it feel more illicit and therefore more pleasurable.

Before my mysterious eye attack, I had been preoccupied and slightly bored, planning what I was going to say, distracted this way and that by what I had to do later. Now I was noticing peoples' lips, and not just noticing them, but fascinated by them, still a little scared, but awake. My hands were shaking slightly which meant I wasn't making any of this up. (Writing this down it sounds like I was stoned. I was not.). Also it felt like everyone was an animal dressed in clothing. Which of course we were, I thought, self-assuredly.

It was thrilling to be in my own private body in class, not distracted or self-absorbed. What could be more mundane then going around a table describing what you are working on? What could be more thrilling than thinking you're going to have a stroke, not having a stroke, and then being fascinated with your own body next to the bodies of others? Now that is a good time to describe what you are working on.

Now I had a different worry: what if my altered perception went away? Because by then I was thinking, *I can use this*. Maybe *this* could be what I am working on for my dissertation.

There's a *Seinfeld* episode where Jerry and George have an idea about a show (which turns out to be about the characters' lives, the show we're watching). George says (I'm paraphrasing), *It's a show about nothing*. And Jerry says, "*Well it's got to be about something*." And George says, "*Nothing*!" I was having that conversation with myself.

"This is my dissertation," my own voice was saying aloud in my head. "What?" my head asked my voice. "What's *this*?" "This feeling," I whispered. "That's it?" my head was saying. "It can't be just a feeling!"

It was almost my turn to talk. "Avi, what are you working on?" Dr. Schubert asked me. I sat there for a moment wondering whether I should lie by telling the truth about what I *was working on*. Instead I told the class about my non-stroke experience. People smiled and waited to see how it would relate. Schubert had stuck the nub of his pen in the ridge of his glasses so that it stuck out like an erection. I thought that was a good sign.

I attempted to theorize on the spot. "What the teacher is feeling and thinking may determine his students experience just as much or more than any content he intends to teach. Fifty percent of how we experience life is non-verbally."[1] The class stared at me blankly. I remember something Brene Brown (2010) said in a Ted Talk, that storytelling is data with a soul. I said that aloud. I launched into another story with the class, about how in 4th grade math, I was pressing my lips up and down my arm, because I liked the saltiness of my skin on my mouth. My math teacher Mr. Putman had pointed me out, and said, "Look at him." And then, remarkably he started singing. "I love my-SELF, I LOVE myself." The grad class loved that story. The story played better than the idea. I almost sounded like Seinfeld telling it. Was that a good thing? I was a grad student trying to write a dissertation in Curriculum Studies not some stand-up comedian trying to make people laugh about what it feels like to be in school.

Schubert suggested that this could make a good study. What I wondered —my salty arm? He said something about narrative inquiry and Dewayne Huebner's (2008) question *what might transpire,* Merleau-Ponty's (2015) phenomenology, Philip Jackson's (1989) book about the mimetic versus the transformative teacher, and that 150 years ago Rousseau (1762/2013) talked about the concept of *losing time* (at least I knew one of the references!), not to mention Maxine Greene's (2000) notion of *becoming* and Jerome McDonald's (1995) classroom experience as a religious experience. Had I read William James *Varieties of Religious Experience* (1902/2016)? *You should* he said.

It was mildly disappointing to know that I was writing about was not strictly original. Then again I had have some needed sources. Mostly, I thought—*what a field!*—where what is divergent and outside our usual frame may relate it untold ways. That night I wrote the narrative of a 5-minute passing period:

The bell rings. I am once again thrust against the throngs of nameless people. I have the usual martyred, waking dream that I am the only human walking amongst machines. The opposite is true, though. The kids are more human since they are younger. They're changing more than I am. Chances are, they will live longer too.

I'm hungry. The thing to do is have a bag of Sun Chips from room 372. Administrator offices, with their leftovers (chips, bagels, fruit, juice cups, even bacon) from meetings are perfect for a secret snack. If I walk in on one side and leave out the other, it will be like I was never there. It's when I start thinking about class that I start thinking about all those essays I haven't read.

Each day, they make the commute back home with me; each day, they stay in the bag. I counter this negativity with something I recently read from Bill Ayers [2016], the former weathermen turned preschool teacher turned professor turned mentor, organizer, writer, renowned speaker extraordinaire: stop waiting for the day when all of the conditions of your life are perfect and get down to the work. Ok fine, but first chips.

A bunch of thoughts bombard me at once. Don't forget to get your mom something for her birthday. Be more sensitive about students' nicknames. Little Greeny might not like being called Little Greeny. Is being Bill Ayers as fun as it seems? You should eat less gluten. also think about the tumor removed from my neck 15 years ago, and my daughter's missing tooth from the time her stroller flipped over. I worry that I haven't accomplished enough. I wonder whether or not I've zipped up my fly. I do a fly-check, because with tasks that happen sequentially it's easy to forget zipping one's fly.

I anxiously walk past my old classroom—the one without windows, in which my class lobbied successfully for the school to paint the walls yellow. They also researched how uncomfortable desks are. Which is how I wound up with beanbags in my room for a couple of years, until the school deemed that they didn't meet the fire code. It would be lovely to take a nap, I think. I walk down the hall to my next class. I am hyper aware of looking at students and being looked at by them. I think about this Eudora Welty story where this character says that the most amazing thing in the entire world is the human face. She's right. It pleases me to greet the students I know and like. They smile or wave hello and we move on, hurled inexorably forward by the inevitability of the next thing.

The hundreds of students I don't know fill me with wonder. I want to sing: "Look at all the people. Where do they all belong?" I am, I realize, again and again, addicted to attention, to the mere possibility of an interaction. I am always managing how much to come out of my skin and how much to stay folded in it. I walk past rm. 348, halfway there to my next class. The clockwork of the day momentarily disintegrates when you encounter people you know but then harshly clicks back into step as you walk on by. (Lessing, 2012)

THE PATH IS THE GOAL

The heart of my dissertation emerged from my nonstroke experience. I wrote a fictional autobiographical narrative describing one day from the perspective of the teacher. It focussed on the visceral, on the connection between the mental and the kinesthetic, the physical and the emotional, the academic and the social. I wrote about all the ways a teacher is distracted and tries to bring his attention back, or sadly, how it stays turned away. Here (Lessing, 2012) is a different hallway scene:

> I head out into the long hallway, which is getting filled from end to end. I'm stuck in the hallway, amongst the masses, the sludge, here comes the painful anonymous feeling you have in an airport. This is where I live a good portion of my life. Students graduate after 4 years, but teachers are caught in the Sisyphus-like act of repeatedly teaching the same thing over and over. Most students walk with their head on a swivel looking side to side. Most teachers walk with their heads down or straight ahead. It's the difference between having a social life at school and having a job to do. Over the tops of the students' heads, some ways down the hall, I see Ben Tucker approaching. Great reputation. Martin, the department head, calls him the best practitioner in the department. Like Martin, he wears khakis and teaches AP English. And like me, he teaches American Studies. What's unique about Ben is that his students blog. And second semester seniors can call him by his first name. He has got unit plans for stuff he doesn't even teach but *hopes to* some day; I've just begun to wrap my head around why a unit plan is necessary in the first place. Bet his evaluations are immaculate.
>
> "Hey Avi," he says and keeps walking. I feel myself subject to automated replies, practiced physical gestures, the mindless route from one place to the next. Everything is predictably dead. I've never been able to figure out why sometimes I have energy in school and other moments my brain feels so limited, scrunched, and incapable of an original thought that I can barely see past my dull, grey, patterned, monotonous thoughts. Seen from afar, I must look like one of those Hassidic types praying by the Wailing Wall, except I'm not praying to god. I'm talking to myself.

I find that most writing about education is prescriptive. We lack simple descriptions of the individual moments as teachers and students experience them; or conversely, as so often is the case, how we are not present, preoccupied, worried, elsewhere. Because if you can recognize the moments where your attention wanders, you have the possibility of paying attention in a more substantial way. Being present or self-aware partly means becoming aware of all the times we are not.

There are those moments in teaching and learning like my nonstroke when the whole room changes, when the feeling changes. Where it feels like something is happening or about to happen. You might meet someone in a new way or catch something in the air that leads to a real insight, or meet yourself in an entirely new way. I am convinced creating a curriculum that values, welcomes, and even encourages these moments may transcend the curriculum of points or targets, and impact us greatly in ways that are difficult to measure. They are turning points that we may leverage for big learnings. For instance, Fyodor Dostoevsky (1868) describes how this kind of moment inspires his writing: "in my head and in my soul many artistic conceptions flash and make themselves felt. But they only flash and what's needed is a full embodiment."

I want to think carefully about how to open up these kinds of experiences in school and how we may embody them fully. When I am in the classroom and my perception brightens, my thoughts are not so crowded anymore, my head is less dull and I can even forget for a second that I am supposed to be in my role: teaching, multiasking, urging, admonishing, checking, scoring, an so forth. Out of nowhere an all-around awareness sometimes come to the fore. It makes you want to look more closely with your eyes. It is a rare affordance in school. Where you know what matters most is what's occurring now. Such brightened perception can only make you more of a resource to your students. Like my mom said if you can stay present and not freak out, you can be anyone in those moments, more than a teacher, or maybe less, the cleaning lady, a body meeting another body, someone truly *in loco- parentis.*

The current educational landscape belies such hopes. It seems a foregone conclusion that our task tilts entirely toward achievement, instead of experience (as if they were separate!). Talking about experience is now an almost forgotten retro theory of education from the 70s. What is visceral or experiential gets dismissed as a distraction from work, as opposed to the gateway towards something potentially transformative.

THE VISCERAL ETHNOGRAPHER

My cousin is a political scientist. A couple of years ago, he invited me to a party that concluded a conference he attended. I was the only one dancing, except for this other anthropologist who researches prison gangs in El Salvador. We danced playful and mockingly, communicating who-knows-what through our movements. He started calling me the Visceral Ethnographer. I did not know what that meant (I do not think he did either). But I liked the implications: to examine how bodies interact in a space, how our physical, primordial reactions impact one another. What if you could actually understand someone else's actions on such an essential level? I rushed up to my cousin to tell him the good news: I was now into visceral ethnography.

"That's not an actual field," he said.

My cousin always teases me that I do not teach content. I tell him the point of teaching is in the interaction of the human beings in the room. We have *google* for content. He says to me that students still need to learn a discipline; they need to learn *something*. Sure, I say, but we have spent the last 100 years almost entirely focused on the something instead of the *somebody*. We were having the same usual argument but this time I cut him off with a visceral dance move.

MORE NOTES ON THE VISCERAL

A colleague and I were talking about theater. She was saying plays should be like concerts, they should make us want to dance. I have been thinking about that in education: what would a curriculum look like that inspires us to want to dance or sing?

If we want to go beyond memorized material towards memorable experiences, we have to find ways for ourselves and our students to be more embodied—not just as an abstraction, but as real observable phenomena. Other surprisingly practical and observable questions we might be interested include: What is our physical proximity to students? Do we sit behind our desks or sit amongst them? Who do we look at and who do our eyes stray from?

STUDENT IMPRESSIONS OF THE VISCERAL

I asked my students once that question, to make it less abstract. What is the feeling you have when you walk in the room? Here is what they wrote:

> I feel far away from everyone particularly today my mind is wandering and I'm sleepy. I want to be home. But not home. My house feels so empty when my parents aren't there. It's a new feeling. I thought I would like it more but I don't. I want them there. This class feels like home. Only on certain days.
>
> There always seems a substantial physical distance between teacher and students. Unless I'm in the first row I always seem to further away than I am. And if I am in the front sometime I think that I may get in the way. It's not super pronounced, but it's noticeable.
>
> For me, the school day is most like a dream. I feel like I'm outside looking in.

A QUICK SAMPLING OF WAYS THE VISCERAL COULD TAKE SHAPE

Examples of the visceral curriculum: (1) Project that gets students embodied: (they can embody a viewpoint, a method, or another person). (2) Anything brings students and teacher inward, that is, reflective writing, meditation, drawing, (3) Any experience that jars students out of normalcy, for example, you come to class in costume or someone has a laugh attack in class. (4) Pair up student who have never spoken to each other and have them partner up and tell a story about themselves to each other (you can use the brilliant Anna Deavere Smith (2001) method and have them repeat it back to each other as if they were the other person).

I REMEMBER

The same year I had Mr. Allison for English, I had Mr. Flatt for Geometry. He wore khkaki pants and button downs, with the collars spread over the sweater, 80s style. I sat in the back row terrified to be called on, completely anonymous. Mr. Flatt stayed at the front of the class smirking. Even now, I remember him as always being at a distance. I never knew the right answer and so I was cut off from having any kind of experience, except a shaming one. The kids who knew the answer predictably enjoyed the class. But for me, he was a remote figure and remembering him caused me shame for a long time after his class was done. In math, I dropped down a level every year.

Now 25 years later, I am an English teacher. I started a Social and Emotional Learning (SEL) pilot program at my school. But like all human beings, I am still negotiating and enlarging my capacity to be more present, less distracted, and more aware, so that my students can have more powerfully embodied experiences. As my mentor told me once: "There's always a feeling in every room. Doesn't mean that it's always positive." It is true, I think. I remember both well.

NOTE

1. Turns out scientists think the number is closer to 80.

REFERENCES

Ayers, W. (2016). *Demand the impossible!: A radical manifesto*. Chicago, IL: Haymarket Books.

Brown, B. (2010, June). *The power of vulnerability*. Speech presented at Ted Talk, Houston, Texas.

Dostoevsky, F. (1868, January 12). [Letter to Apollon Maikov].

Greene, M. (2000). *Releasing the imagination: Essays on education, the arts, and social change*. San Francisco, CA: Jossey-Bass.

Huebner, D. E., Pinar, W. F., & Hillis, V. (2008). *The lure of the transcendent: Collected essays by Dwayne E. Huebner*. New York, NY: Routledge.

Hughes, J. D. (Director). (1986). *Ferris Bueller's day off* [Motion picture]. United States: Paramount Pictures.

Jackson, P. W. (1989). *The practice of teaching*. New York, NY: Teachers College Press.

James, W. (2016). *The varieties of religious experience: A study in human nature: Being the Gifford Lectures on natural religion delivered at Edinburgh in 1901–1902*. United States: CreateSpace Independent Publishing Platform. (Original work published 1902)

Lessing, A. D. (2012). *Into me you see* (Unpublished doctoral dissertation). University of Illinois, Chicago.

Merleau-Ponty, M., & Smith, C. (2015). *Phenomenology of perception*. London, England: Forgotten Books.

Rousseau, J. (2013). *Emile*. Mineola, NY: Dover. (Original work published 1762)

Salinger, J. D. (2014). *The catcher in the rye: A novel*. New York, NY: Little, Brown and Company.

Smith, A. D. (2001). *Talk to me: Travels in media and politics*. New York, NY: Anchor Books.

CHAPTER 7

INTERSECTING RACE, LANGUAGE, AND IDENTITY

Toward a Sensuous Curriculum of Investment

Awad Ibrahim
University of Ottawa

> The word in language is half someone else's. It becomes "one's own" only when the speaker populates it with his own intention, his own accent, when he appropriates the word, adapting it to his own semantic and expressive intention. Prior to this moment of appropriation, the word does not exist in a neutral and impersonal language (it is not, after all, out of a dictionary that a speaker gets his words!) but rather it exists in other people's mouths, in other people's concrete contexts, serving other people's intentions: it is from there that one must take the word and make it one's own.
>
> Mikhail M. Bakhtin (as cited in Toohey, 2000)

A different version of this chapter appeared in Ibrahim, A. (2011). When life is off da hook: Hip-Hop identity and identification, BESL, and the pedagogy of pleasure. In C. Higgins (Ed.), *Negotiating the self in another language: Identity formation in a globalized world* (pp. 221–238). Berlin, Germany: Mouton de Gruyter.

Sensuous Curriculum:
Politics and the Senses in Education, pp. 115–134

Curriculum, it seems, has different interests for different people, especially when it comes to psychic and emotional investment. Here, one invests where one sees oneself mirrored. Referencing a published study (Ibrahim, 2011, 2014), my aim in this chapter is to discuss fragments from that study using the concepts of "investment," "sensuous," and "sensuality." The study focuses on a group of continental African youth who enter, so to speak, a "rhizome of Blackness," where Blackness is not one but multiple categories with multiple meanings and frames of reference. The end result, I will show, is, first, learning Black English as a Second Language (BESL) (instead of so-called "standard English" or ESL) and, second, taking up and investing into Hip-Hop cultural identity, which these young people access in and through Black popular culture. I will offer, in conclusion, a terse discussion on what I am calling a 'sensual curriculum of investment.'

INVESTMENT AND SENSUALITY: THE STORY OF A LANGUAGE LEARNING–TAKE I

Little learning, if any, happens outside that space of *mé*tissage (Ibrahim, 2014), that hybrid space where the micro and the macro meet, where the deeply individual, subjective, and affective meet the broader social forces, and where power and social differences (be it race, gender, sexuality, etc.) meet investment. To address the latter notion of investment, we need to ask: why do we learn what we learn and "why a learner can sometimes speak and other times remains silent" (Peirce, 1995, p. 11)? By way of answering, we need to start with certain premises: that the individual does not exist in a social vacuum, that we do not choose our life chances (i.e., where we are born, to whom we are born, our race, gender, abilities, etc.), that these life chances are sometimes inequitably distributed and thus either open or close possibilities for learning, that we are forever marked by history, that our identities are social as much as they are subjectively individual (if not more), that learning is deeply contextual (i.e., happens in a time, a place and between actors), and that learning is conscious as much as it is deeply affective, sensuous, and unconscious.

In a classic article linking social identity, power relations, and language learning, Bonny Norton Peirce (1995) foregrounds "the role of language as constitutive of and constituted by a language learner's social identity" (p. 13). That is to say, language is "the place where actual and possible forms of social organization and their likely social and political consequences are defined and contested ... [and it is] the place where our sense of ourselves, our subjectivity, is constructed" (Weedon, as cited in Peirce, 1995, p. 15). Here, the subject and his/her subjectivity have three defining characteristics: (1) they are multiple and non-unitary; (2) they are sites of struggle and contestation; and (3) they are forever changing, unstable and "rhizomatic" (Ibrahim, 2014). Moreover, as much as learning is contextual, Peirce (1995) explains, humans are endowed with human agency, where, dependent on the context, we position, perform, recite, and utter ourselves differently in different contexts. These different utterances of our subjectivity make us-subject multiple, contradictory and a site of struggle.

Because of this reconceptualization of social identity and subjectivity, Peirce (1995) contends, we need to decouple and rescue sensuality and investment from the psychological notion of motivation. For Peirce, the psychological approach to motivation, by and large, is linear, acontextual, ahistorical, and does not deal directly deal with power relations. Investment, on the other hand, starts by situating the subject in a space, time and history. The subject is always endowed with agency and desire. It is this agency and desire that determines what we learn, why we learn what we learn and what symbolic and material capitals (Bourdieu, 1977) we access through the act of learning. As I will show below, we invest into that which is hitherto unattainable and/or that which is meaningful to us. In becoming meaningful, the site of our investment has to be appealing; that is, it has to become emotionally, psychically, and affectively a site of identification: a mirror through which we see ourselves reflected. As such, it is important to note, the notion of investment is an umbrella term where the conscious act of learning is meshed with the deeply affective, sensual, and unconscious. To explain, in a second language learning context, for example, learning a second language is determined not by grammar and syntax, but by asking: why am I learning a second language, what do I want to do with it, and where does it serve me? In this sense, learning a second language is an affective—not to say sensual—act: the more we sense and feel the immediacy of language (i.e., its utility and impact in our everyday struggle for voice, jobs, and gaining our rights to speak) the more we invest and hence the more competent we become in the said language.

INVESTMENT AND SENSUALITY: THE STORY OF A LANGUAGE LEARNING—TAKE II

The act of language learning, namely learning English as a Second Language (ESL), as we shall see in the rest of this chapter, is turned into a symbolic act of identity negotiation and translation; an act of desire, investment, identity, and identification; an act which forms and simultaneously performs a subject formation project where Blackness is central. Examining the intersection of race, identity, and language learning, the chapter is an exploration of the process of *becoming Black*. The chapter is anchored on two premises. The first is that, in North America, youths from 11 to 20 years old do not learn ESL inside the ESL classroom. This is not to suggest that youths do not learn at all in the ESL classroom. We know they do. I wish, however, to argue that youths will go extensively beyond what we teach in our ESL classrooms to learn everyday idioms and the conventional ways of using them. After all, as Bakhtin argues, it is not out of a dictionary that a speaker/learner gets her words. The second premise of the chapter is that youths' gendered, sexualized, abled, classed, and racialized social identities are directly implicated in the ESL learning process. Indeed, they are its foundations (cf. Ibrahim, 2016, 2014, 2006; Morgan, 1998; Norton & Toohey, 2004), and no learning would be made personal, Bakhtin argues, unless the learner *populates* the word with his/her own intentions, his/her own accent; hence, appropriating the word and adapting it to his/her own semantic and expressive intentions and affective, sensual investment.

The chapter argues that a group of French-speaking immigrant and refugee continental African youths who are attending an urban Franco-Ontarian high school in southwestern Ontario, Canada, enters *a social imaginary*—a discursive space in which they are already imagined, constructed, and thus treated as Blacks by hegemonic discourses and groups. This imaginary is directly implicated in whom they identify with (Black North America), which in turn influences what and how they learn linguistically and culturally. They learn Black Stylized English (BSE), a subcategory of Black English (BE), which they access in Hip-Hop culture and Rap lyrical and linguistic styles. For them, BE becomes as much a site of language learning as a symbolic space of identification, investment, and desire; and the act of learning is no longer a neutral act. In fact, it raises a number of critical questions. First, why would continental African youths *need* and *want* to learn, appropriate, re-produce, and re-perform these *symbolic systems* (Bourdieu, 1991), and, second, what does it mean for a Black ESL learner to acquire Black English as a Second Language (BESL)? That is, at a time when North American Blackness is governed by how negatively it is located in a race-conscious society (Dixson & Rousseau, 2006; Simmons, 2016), what symbolic, cultural, pedagogical, and identity investments would learners have in locating themselves politically and racially at the margin of representation?

By *symbolic system,* I am referring to a set of norms, rules, and regulations that are expressly operating together to create an entity, a form, a mode, a structure, or what Foucault (Rabinow, 1984) calls "discourse"—an ensemble of discursive formations or frameworks forming and re/transforming who we are and determining what we can and must say (Hall, 1996). They are symbolic because they are misrecognized or least visible (Bourdieu, 1991); yet, they constitute the deep and infrastructures of any material system. In a dialectic sense, they are constituents of and at the same time constituting these infrastructures. Put otherwise, symbolic systems need material systems—what Bourdieu (1991) calls champs ("fields")—in order to exist and function, however, they also constitute the very grounds upon which the material system depends and indeed where the latter expresses itself. I have an identity, for example, but my identity would not exist outside the *linguistic field* where it expresses itself. This is why, as Peirce suggested above, language is where subjectivity and agency are both formed and performed.

Language, it is worth adding, is where we express our feelings, who we are or what we have become, and where we invest our desires. Here, language is not, and has never been, just an instrument of communication, as I argued elsewhere (Ibrahim, 2014). It is also where power is formed and performed based on race, gender, sexuality, and social-class identity. In what follows, I first explore my research and its methodology and findings and, then, offer a conclusion on the need for what I am calling: sensual curriculum of investment.

HANGING OUT: ETHNOGRAPHY OF PERFORMANCE AND MARIE-VICTORIN[1]

The research for this chapter constitutes part of a larger critical ethnographic research[2] project I conducted (Ibrahim, 2014, 2011) in 2007 and 2011. In both, I asked the following questions: (1) First, what are the roads taken by African youths in their journey of integration in the Canadian society, the journey of *becoming Black*?; (2) What is the role of race and racism in their identity formation?; (3) How are continental African youths positioned and constructed in and out of school?; 4) What are the implications of this construction in youths' social identity formation?; and (5) What are the outcomes of this journey?

I developed a methodological approach which I call *ethnography of performance* to understand how African youths in Ontario perform identities, desires, and investments in and through the complex semiological languages of their dress, walk, and talk. Unlike Denzin (2003) who uses the term "performance ethnography" to analyze "text," my text is an actual Black body (or socially perceived as such). This critical ethnographic study of performance allows access as researchers to our research subjects' inner-identity, what they think and desire, and how they long to represent themselves and to be represented. In other words, identities, I am contending, are best accessed in and through observing what people do and perform on the surface of their bodies. And to have a complete picture of our research subjects' identities, if ever this is possible, we need to follow them extensively in different places, at different times, and over extended period of time; and ask them to verbalize and reflect upon their own performances/actions.

At both times of the research, I was well acquainted with the school and its population since I had carried out research there for almost two years in the later 1990s. With permission from the school administration, I began visiting the school in 2007 and then in 2011 to *hang out*[3] with African students at least once a week, and in some cases, two or three times for almost six months in 2007 and 2 months in 2011. I took the role of a participant-observer, keeping regular field notes. Having determined what they could offer to my research, I chose for extensive observation sixteen students—10 boys and 6 girls—between the ages of 14 and 20. Constituting part of my purposeful sampling (Denzin, 2003), these participants are chosen as a representative sample based on their gender, age, being active, being academic, social or sport-oriented, and so forth (see Ibrahim, 2014 for a full discussion). The girls were Somali-speakers from Somalia and Djibouti. Of the 10 boys, 6 were Somali-speakers—from Somalia and Djibouti, 2 Senegalese, 1 Ethiopian and 1 Togolese. I observed them in and out of school. With the consent of students and their parents, I interviewed them, individually or in-groups, for an 1 to 3 hours, at the school or at their residences. Interviews were either in English or French; the majority, however, were in French. I also videotaped and in two occasions handed over the tape recorders to students to capture their interactions among themselves when I was not present. I attended soirées, plays, basketball games, and graduations, and I was delighted to be invited to their residences. I transcribed and translated the interviews and some of the videotapes, and analyzed the data by grouping them by theme, category and subject.

The School Context

Marie-Victorin (MV) is a small intermediate and high school of approximately 400 students from various ethnic, racial, cultural, religious, and linguistic backgrounds. Though it is a French-language school, the language spoken by students in the school corridors and hallways was predominately English; Arabic, Somali, and Farsi were also spoken at other times. In both periods of research, I attended classes at MV, talked to students, and observed curricular and extracurricular activities two or three times per week. Being the only Black adult—with the exception of one Black counselor—and being a displaced subject, a refugee, and an African, gave me a certain familiarity with the students' experiences. I was able to connect with different age and gender groups through a range of activities, initially hanging out with the students and later playing sports with various groups. I was also approached by these students for both guidance and academic help. Because of my deep involvement in the student culture, at times my status as a researcher was forgotten, and the line between the students and myself became blurred; clearly, we shared a safe space of comfort that allowed us to open up, speak, and engage freely.

Notably, MV had a high immigrant population at the times of this research. In fact, students who were or had parents who were born outside Canada made up 30–40% of the entire school population. Among them, continental Africans constituted the majority. MV administration emphasized the theme of unity within this multicultural and multiethnoracial population. The slogan that the school advertised was *unité dans la diversité* (unity in diversity). This discourse of unity, however, had little material bearing on the students' material lives, as we shall see, and it was the Frenchness of the school that seemed to be the cultural and linguistic capital (Bourdieu, 1991) of its promotion. And given its symbolic value, most African youths come to MV with a highly valued European linguistic norm of French: *le français parisien* (Parisian French).

Participants

My research participants formed part of a growing continental francophone African population in Franco-Ontarian schools, whose numbers have grown exponentially since the beginning of the 1990s. The participants varied in their length of stay in Canada, their legal status (some were immigrants, but the majority were refugees), gender, class, age, and their linguistic and national backgrounds. They came from places as diverse as the Democratic Republic of Congo (formerly Zaïre), Djibouti, Gabon, Senegal, Somalia, South Africa, and Togo. With no exception, all of the African students in MV were at least trilingual, speaking English, French, and their mother tongues, with various postcolonial histories of language learning and degrees of fluency in each language.

The research tells the stories of a group of continental Francophone African youth and the formation of their social identity in an urban, French-language high school in southwestern Ontario. Besides their gendered and racialized experience, their youth and refugee status was vital in their *moments of identification*, that is, where and how they saw themselves reflected in the mirror of their society (cf. Bhabha, 1994). Put differently, once in North America, I contend, these youths were faced with a *social imaginary* in which they were already Blacks. This social imaginary was directly implicated in how and with whom they identified, which, in turn, influenced what they learned, linguistically and culturally. What they did learn is Black Stylized English (BSE), which they accessed in and through

Black popular culture. They learned by taking up and repositing the Rap linguistic and musical genre and, in different ways, acquiring and rearticulating the Hip-Hop cultural identity.

Black Stylized English

BSE is a subcategory of Black English (BE), what Geneva Smitherman refers to as *Black talk* (2000), which has its own grammar, morphology and syntax. BSE, on the other hand, refers to ways of speaking that do not depend on a full mastery of the language. It banks more on ritual expressions such as *whassup, whadap, whassup* [what is happening] *my Nigga*, and *yo, yo homeboy,* which are performed habitually and recurrently in Rap. These rituals, I explain elsewhere are more an expression of politics, moments of identification, and desire than they are of language or of mastering the language *per se* (Ibrahim, 2014). It is a way of saying, "I too am Black" or "I too desire and identify with Blackness."

Here, Black popular culture refers to films, newspapers, magazines, and more importantly music, such as rap, reggae, pop, and rhythm and blues (R&B). By *Hip-Hop* I am referring to an umbrella term that refers to everything from music, to clothing choices, attitudes, language, and an approach to culture and cultural artifacts positing and collaging them in an unsentimental fashion (see especially Chang, 2005; Alim, Ibrahim, & Pennycook, 2009). More specifically, I use Hip-Hop to describe a way of dressing, walking, and talking. The *dress* refers to the myriad shades and shapes of the latest fly gear: high-top sneakers, bicycle shorts, chunky jewelry, baggy pants, and polka-dotted tops (Rose, 1991, p. 227). The *walk* usually means moving the fingers simultaneously with the head and the rest of the body while walking. The *talk*, however, is BSE. In patterning these behaviors, African youth enter the realm of becoming Black. In sum, becoming Black is a *subject-formation project* (i.e., the process and the space within which subjectivity is formed) that is produced in and simultaneously produced by the process of language learning—BESL learning in this case. More specifically, becoming Black means learning BESL; yet the very process of BESL learning produces the epiphenomenon of becoming Black.

With regard to performances involving BESL, I saw almost no difference among the students in 2007 and 2011. This confirmed the primary tenet of my early research, which was that, once in North America, continental African youths enter a specific *social imaginary*, where already constructed, imagined, and positioned as Blacks. Their positionality is as much their treatment by hegemonic discourses and dominant groups, as other groups of color or Black Canadians whose in-group acknowledgements at once reaffirm their inclusion as Blacks in Canada and the oppressed and marginalized positionality their Blackness engenders. This space of (mostly subconscious) psychic formation does not acknowledge the differences in the students' ethnicities, languages, nationalities, and cultural identities. Elsewhere (Ibrahim, 2011), I quoted Fanon (1967), as he sums up it brilliantly, writing about himself as a Black *Antillais* coming to the metropolitan center of Paris: "I am given no chance, I am overdetermined from without. I am the slave not of the "idea" that others have of me but of my own appearance" (p. 116).

The students' BSE performances confirm that continental African youth find themselves in a racially conscious society that, wittingly or unwittingly and through fused social mechanisms such as racist representations, asks them to racially fit somewhere. To fit somewhere signifies choosing or becoming aware of one's own being, which is partially reflected in one's language practice. Choosing, however, is also a question of agency, which itself is governed and disciplined by social conditions (Ortner, 2006). For example, to be Black in a racially conscious society, like the Euro-Canadian and U.S. societies, means that one is expected to be Black, act Black, and so be the marginalized *other* (Alim & Smitherman, 2012; Shaw-Taylor & Tuch, 2007).

SIGNIFYING BESL LEARNING: TAKING UP HIP-HOP AS A SUBJECT FORMATION PROJECT

Except in Quebec, the English language is normally the medium of everyday interaction in Canada. This creates a situation where African youth would want to learn English rapidly. Popular culture, especially television, as well as friendship and peer pressure are three mechanisms that hasten the speed of learning the language (Ibrahim, 2014). The African students felt peer pressure particularly in their early days at the school when they were denigrated for not speaking English. The pressure was even greater since, as Heller (2006) has explained, Franco-Ontarian students use English in their everyday interactions, especially outside class. If African students want to participate in school activities, they have no option but to learn English.

Making friends, and even learning English, is influenced by the popular imaginary, projected through the dominant source of representation: television. I asked students in all of the interviews, *"Où est-ce que vous avez appris votre anglais?"* (Where did you learn English?). *"Télévision,"* they all responded. However, within this *télévision* is a particular representation—Black popular culture—seems to *interpellate*[4] (Althusseur, 1971) African youths' identity investment, formation and identification. Because

African youths at first have few African Canadian/American friends, they access Black cultural identities and Black linguistic practice through Black popular culture, especially rap music video-clips, television programs, and Black cinema. When Najat (14, F, Djibouti)[5] was queried about the most recent movies she had seen, she responded:

> Najat: I don't know, I saw *Waiting to Exhale* and I saw what else I saw, I saw Swimmer, and I saw Jumanji; so wicked, all the movies. I went to *Waiting to Exhale*wid my boyfriend and I was like 'men are rude' [laughs].
>
> Awad: Oh believe me I know I know.
>
> Najat: And den he [her boyfriend] was like "no women are rude." I was like we're like fighting you know and joking around. I was like, and de whole time like [laughs], and den when de woman burns the car, I was like "go girl!" You know and all the women are like "go girl!" you know? And den de men like khhh. I'm like "I'm gonna go get me a pop corn" [laughs] (individual interview, English).

Najat's response is of particular interest for two reasons. First, it shows the influence of Black English in the use of *de*, *den*, *dat*, and *wicked* as opposed to, respectively, *the*, *then*, *that*, and *really really good*. Second, it shows that youths' social subjectivities, embedded in history, culture, and memory influence what they read and how they interpret it. For example, Najat's reading of *Waiting to Exhale* was interpellated by her race and gender identities. She identified with the Black/woman in burning her husband's car and clothes. Clearly, this is a demonstrative moment identification and identity and sensual investment.

The following is another example (a videotaped moment) demonstrating the impact of Black popular culture on African students' lives, identification, and identities. Just before a focus group interview I had with the boys, *Electric Circus*, a local Canadian television music and dance program that plays mostly, if not exclusively, Black music (Hip-Hop, reggae, soul, and R&B) began. "*Silence!*" one boy exclaimed in French. The boys started to listen attentively to the music and to watch the different fashions of the young people on the program. After the show, the boys' code switched between French, English, and Somali as they exchanged observations on the best music, the best dance, and the cutest girl. Rap and Hip-Hop music and the corresponding dress were at the top of their list.

These moments of identification point to the process of identity formation which is, in turn, implicated in the linguistic norm to be populated (using Bakhtin's term) and invested in. A significant aspect to note about identification is that it works over a period of time and at the subconscious level. Omer (18, M, Ethiopia), in the following excerpt, addresses the different ways in which African youths are influenced by their identification with Black representations.

> Black Canadian youths are influenced by the Afro-Americans. You watch for hours, you listen to Black music, you watch Black comedy, *Mr. T.*,[8] the *Rap City*. There you will see singers who dress in particular ways. You see, so. (individual interview, French)

Mukhi (19, M, Djibouti) explored identification by arguing that:

> We identify ourselves more with the Blacks of America. But, this is normal; this is genetic. We can't, since we live in Canada, we can't identify ourselves with Whites or country music, you know [laughs]. We are going to identify ourselves, on the contrary, with people of our color, who have our life style, you know (group interview, French).

Here, Mukhi's identification with Blackness is clearly pronounced. For Mukhi and all the students I spoke to, this identification is linked to their inability to relate to dominant groups, the public spaces they occupy, and their cultural forms and norms. Alternatively, Black popular culture emerged not only as a site for identification, but also as a space for language learning.

(B)ESL AND THE ECONOMY OF POPULATION

For African youths, Rap/Hip-Hop was one site that emerged as more than just a cultural site of entertainment. It was also an influential *sensual curriculum* site of *investment* and language learning. Yet, importantly, Hip-Hop/Rap was more recurrent in the boys' narratives than in the girls', which raises the question of the role of gender in the process of identification and learning. The boys, for instance, seemed to invest substantially in this economy of Hip-Hop and Gangsta Rap language and style, which surfaced on their bodies and in their linguistic style. This is what I am calling an *economy of population*, an economy of identity, linguistic, cultural, sensual and affective investment, where no investment is haphazard and most of it takes place subconsciously. The following excerpts are two of the many occasions on which students performed their investment in Black North America through the re/citation of Rap linguistic styles.[6]

Sam: One two, one two, mic check. A'ait [alright], a'ait, a'ait.

Juma: This is the rapper, you know wha 'm meaning? You know wha 'm saying?

Sam: Mic micmic; mic check. A'ait you wonna test it? Ah, I've the microphone you know; a'ait.

Sam: [laughs] I don't rap man, c'mon give me a break. [laughs] Yo! A'aita'ait you know, we just about to finish de tape and all dat. Respect to my main man [pointing to me]. So, you know, you know wha 'm mean, 'm just represen'in Q7. One love to Q7 you know wha 'm mean and all my friends back to Q7... Stop the tapin boy!

Jamal: Kim Juma, live! Put the lights on. Wordap. [Students talking in Somali] Peace out, wardap, where de book. Jamal 'am outa here.

Shapir: Yo, this is Shapir. I am trying to say peace to all my Niggaz, all my bitches from a background that everybody in the house. So, yo, chill out and this is how we gonna kick it. Bye and with that pie. All right, peace yo.

Sam: A'ait this is Sam represen'in AQA [...] where it's born, represen'in you know wha 'm mean? I wonna say whassup to all my Niggaz, you know, peace and one love. You know wha 'm mean, Q7 represen'in for-ever. Peace! [Rap music]

Jamal: [as a DJ] Crank it man, coming up. [rap music] (group interview, English)

These excerpts are significant for many reasons. First, they demonstrate the influence of BSE, particularly the language of rap: "Respect for my main man," "represen'in Q7," "kick the free style," "peace out, wardap," "am outa here," "I am trying to say peace to all my Niggaz, all my bitches," "so, yo chill out and this is how we gonna kick it," "I wonna say whassup to all my Niggaz," "peace and one love". Second, when Shapir offers "peace to all" his "Niggaz," all his "bitches," he is indeed repossessing the term *Nigga,* a signifier common in Rap/Hip-Hop culture. It is common, for example nowadays, to call a Black friend, especially young people, *Nigga* without its traditional racist connotation. However, Shapir is also using sexist language that exists in Rap (Rose, 1991; Ibrahim, 2000). These forms of sexism have been challenged by female rappers like Queen Latifa and Lil Kim and were critiqued by fellow female and male students. For example, Samira (16, F, Djibouti) expressed her dismay at the sexist language found in some rap lyrics:

> OK, <u>hip-hop</u>, yes I know that everyone likes <u>hip-hop</u>. They dress in a certain way, no? The songs go well. But, they are really really, they have

> expressions like fuck, bitches etc. Sorry, but there is representation. (group interview, French)

The question of representation raised by Samira needs further exploration. Samira is addressing the impact that Hip-Hop expressions might have on the way society at large relates to, consumes, and perceives the Black female body, which in turn influences how it is represented both inside and outside Hip-Hop culture. One may even argue that these narratives, which express a psychic representation and mentality, are in part responsible for Samira's precarious relation with Hip-Hop. Some boys also cited similar language of critique: "Occasionally, rap has an inappropriate language for the life in which we live, a world of violence and all that" (Hassan —17, M, Djibouti—individual interview, French).

In the above excerpts, there are clear indications of Hip-Hop style, where one starts a performance by "checking the mic": "One two, one two, mic check." Then the rapper or the MC either recites an already composed lyric or otherwise "kicks a free style," displaying the spontaneity that characterizes Rap. The rapper begins the public performance by introducing herself or himself with a true or made-up name—"yo this is Shapir"—and thanks her or his "main man," or best friend, who often introduces the rapper to the public. Specific to Gangsta Rap, however, one represents not only oneself but a web of geophysical and metaphorical spaces and collectivities that are demarcated by people and territorial spaces: "represen'in Q7," "a'ait, this is Sam represen'in AQA." At the end of the performance, when the recitation or freestyle is completed, again one thanks the "main man" and "gives peace out" or "shad out" (shout out) to the people.

In its broader semiological sense, Hip-Hop was an influential sensuous curricular site of identification and language learning for the boys, especially Gangsta Rap. Depending on their age, the girls, on the other hand, had an ambivalent relationship to Rap. Although both boys and girls used the same three strategies in learning ESL in general, and BSE in particular, through music: listening, reading and reciting. Jamal, in the above cited extract, for instance, was listening to the tunes and lyrics while reading and following the written text. Acting as a DJ, he then repeated not only the performer's words and expressions but also his accent.[7] The girls also used similar strategies to Jamal's. During a picnic organized by a mixed group of males and females; for example, they listened to music while following the written text and reciting it (complete with accents) along with the singer. The girls' choice of music (e.g., Whitney Houston, Toni Braxton, and other R&B female singers) differed in that it was softer than that chosen by the boys and contained mostly romantic themes.

As I have indicated, for the most part, the older girls/women (16–18 years old) tended to be more eclectic in how they related to Hip-Hop. Their eclecticism was evident in how they dressed and in the language they populated, engaged and learned (Ibrahim, 2003). Their clothing was either elegant middle class, partially Hip-Hop, or traditional, and their learned language was what Nourbese Philip (1991) calls *plain Canadian English*. The younger girls (12–14 years), on the other hand, like the boys, dressed in Hip-Hop style and performed BSE. Nonetheless, I was able to detect three features of BE in both the older and the younger girls' narratives: the absence of the auxiliary be, BE negative concord, and the distributive be (for further details, see Ibrahim, 2014).

PERFORMATIVE LANGUAGE, IDENTIFICATION AND ACTS OF DESIRE

African youths' narratives demonstrate that they were quite volitional in their identification with Blackness and that the process of racialization had directly impacted their choices. As Amani (16, F, Somalia) explains:

> We have to wonder why we try to really follow the model of the Americans who are Black? Because *when you search for yourself, search for identification, you search for someone who reflects you, with whom you have something in common* [italics added]. (group interview, French)

Amani was supported by Mukhi in the following conversation where he reflected on the impact of Rap (as just one among many other Black popular cultural forms) on his life and other lives around him:

> Awad: But do you listen to rap for example? I noticed that there are a number of students who listen to rap eh? Is ...
>
> Sam: It is not just us who listen to rap, everybody listens to rap. It is new.
>
> Awad: But do you think that that influences how you speak, how ...
>
> Mukhi: How we dress, how we speak, how we behave [italics added] (group interview, English).

These linguistic patterns and dress codes that Mukhi is addressing are, on the one hand, accessed and learned by African youths through Black popular culture and, on the other, as I already noted, do not require mastery and fluency. Indeed, they are performative acts of desire and identification. Agreeing with both Mukhi and Amani, Hassan states:

Hassan: Yes yes, African students are influenced by rap and Hip-Hop because they want to, yes, they are influenced probably a bit more because it is the desire to belong may be.

Awad: Belong to what?

Hassan: To a group, belong to a society, to have a model/fashion [he used the term *un modèle*]; you know, the desire to mark oneself, the desire to make, how do I say it? To be part of a rap society, you see. It is like getting into rock and roll or heavy metal. (individual interview, French)

As I argued already, clearly one invests where one sees oneself mirrored. Hassan indicated in an individual interview that it would be awkward to see Blackness allied with rock and roll or heavy metal, as they are socially constructed as White music. On the other hand, he argued emphatically that African youth would have every reason to invest in basketball—constructed as a Black sport—but not hockey, for example.

BY WAY OF CONCLUDING: IDENTITY AND THE SENSUOUS CURRICULUM OF INVESTMENT

> Though they seem to invoke an origin in a historical past with which they continue to correspond, actually identities are about questions of using the resources of history, language, and culture in the process of becoming rather than being: not "who we are" or "where we came from," so much as what we might become, how we have been represented and how that bears on how we might represent ourselves ... not the so-called return to roots but a coming-to-terms-with our "routes." (Hall, 1996, p. 4)

It is these "routes" that I tried to walk through in this chapter. In so doing, I explored the roads taken by African youths in their journey of becoming Black and the outcomes of that journey. Here, Hip-Hop was identified as an influential site of identification and affective investment in African students' processes of becoming Black, which in turn affected what and how they learned. I have argued that the desire on the part of African youths, particularly the boys, to invest in or "populate" basketball is analogously no different from their desire to learn BESL. Thus, creating an economy of population, where learning is neither aimless nor neutral, nor is it without the politics of identity. As I have shown, a second language learner can have a marginalized linguistic norm as a target, depending on who is learning what, why and how. I have also discussed how these youth are becoming

Blacks. Becoming Black, I have argued, is a subject formation project produced by and producing the very process of BESL. To become Black is to become an ethnographer who translates and looks around in an effort to understand what it means to be Black in Canada, for example.

Choosing the margin, then, is simultaneously an act of investment, an expression of desire, and a deliberate counterhegemonic undertaking. Choosing Hip-Hop must be read as a special act of resistance. Historically, Rap/Hip-Hop has been formed as a voice for voicelessness and performed as a prophetic language that addresses silence, the silenced, and the state of being silenced. African youth circulate and form their identities in a social and historical context where everyday racisms, human degradation, and being under the hegemonic gaze are daily occurances. Elsewhere, I have discussed the significance of linking the students' world with their word, their identities with what we teach and how we teach it (Ibrahim, 2014). I have also proposed Hip-Hop as pedagogical sites that can be used in ESL classrooms (Ibrahim, 2004).

Here, I want to take a different turn by offering what I am calling "sensuous curriculum of investment." Through this curriculum, the paper is straddling the fields of literacy/language studies (Peirce, 1995), critical youth studies (Ibrahim & Steinberg, 2014), and critical curriculum studies (Ng-A-Fook, Ibrahim, & Reis, 2016). Situated squarely within the latter critical curriculum studies, sensual curriculum of investment criticalizes (Steinberg, 2014) the very field of curriculum by introducing "sensual" and "investment" to it. Being "critical" does not allow for any curriculum to simply celebrate. It begins with the premise that social products are contextual and historical. As such, proposing Hip-Hop as a site of curriculum does not absolve Hip-Hop from being a hyper masculine space and can even be misogynistic and homophobic. By proposing Hip-Hop as a curriculum site of investment, however, I am arguing that that is where our youth are investing their identities and desires. If we do not engage such a site, then are we not dismissing our students' identities and affective and sensual investment? The end result of such a dismissal is well known, be it drop out, disengagement, and simply finding school boring. By situating sensual curriculum of investment within "criticality" (Steinberg, 2014), I am arguing precisely to engage Hip-Hop not as a site of celebration, but as a social and historical product where our youth (at least in my study) are investing their identities and desire, but that site is open to the beautiful as much as it is open to the ugly, the homophobic, and the sexist. This is why it has to be approached critically.

Sensuous curriculum of investment then begins with the finding of my study, that learning is deeply a sensual act, an act where we invest in where we see ourselves mirrored. Here, the macro power relations and social difference (our race, gender, sexuality, etc.) are an organic and tautological part of what we learn and what we end up populating and investing in. That is to say, we use all our senses when we are engaged with what we are learning; we are driven by an internal drive when we desire to know more; and we have butterfly feelings when we discover something new. Within my study, sensuous curriculum of investment is a call to return and reposition subjectivities and social identities back into language learning mechanisms and techniques and link the cultural, the social, the political, the stylistic, with the linguistic. Central to this repositioning, however, are notions of identification, desire, senses and investment. We are yet to desire "the true word" to be spoken, Paulo Freire (1993) argued, only then can we desire "the world" differently. This is when learning is off da hook: dope, catchy, enticing, attractive, meaningful, sensuous, and sensual ... you got the picture, right?

NOTES

1. All names used in this chapter are pseudonyms.
2. For Simon and Dippo (1986, p. 195), *critical ethnographic research* is a set of activities situated within a project that seeks and works its way towards social transformation. This project is political as well as pedagogical, and who the researcher is and what his or her racial, gender, and class embodiments are necessarily govern the research questions and findings. The project, then, according to Simon and Dippo, is "an activity determined both by real and present conditions, *and* certain conditions still to come which it is trying to bring into being" (p. 196). The assumption underpinning my project was based on the assertion that Canadian society is "inequitably structured and dominated by a hegemonic culture that suppresses a consideration and understanding of why things are the way they are and what must be done for things to be otherwise" (p. 196).
3. Staying somewhere to familiarize oneself with the place, its people, and their ways of "being" in that space. In the school, these sites are informal, such as hallways, the schoolyards, the school steps, the cafeteria, and the gymnasium, where the people in them are comfortable enough to speak their minds.
4. The subconscious ways in which individuals, given their genealogical history and memory, identify with particular discursive spaces and representations and the way this identification subsequently participates in the social formation of the Subject (identity).
5. Each participant's name is followed by his/her age, gender (F = female, M = Male), and country of origin; and each extract is followed by the type of interview (individual or group) and the language in which it was conducted. The following transcription conventions are used:
   underlined text English spoken within French speech or French spoken within English speech
   [ ] Explanation or description of speaker's actions
   [...] Text omitted

6. The participants cited in the extracts are Sam (19, M, Djibouti), Juma (19, M, Senegal), Jamal (18, M, Djibouti), and Shapir (17, M, Somalia).
7. I want to acknowledge here the ongoing debate on sociocultural appropriation and dissemination; that is to say, using the old mantra, of Black innovation and White imitation. These young people are aware of this debate and at the same time, they use it to their advantage. As I show elsewhere (Ibrahim, 2014), part of their becoming Black is precisely becoming aware of this history of how Black culture, language, and musical productions have been misused and outright used to advantage multinational corporations, whose eyes are strictly on how much money they can make. How that is done, and to whose disadvantage is a question that is hardly asked. I explore this debate further in the larger project (see Ibrahim, 2014).

REFERENCES

Alim, A., & Smitherman, G. (2012). *Articulate while Black: Barack Obama, language, and race in the US*. Oxford, England: Oxford University Press.

Alim, S., Ibrahim, A., & Pennycook, A. (2009). *Global linguistic flows: Hip-hop cultures, youth identities, and the politics of language*. London, England & New York, NY: Routledge.

Althusser, L. (1971). *Lenin and philosophy*. London, England: New Left Books.

Bhabha, H. (1994). *The location of culture*. London, England and New York, NY: Routledge.

Bourdieu, P. (1977). The economics of linguistic exchanges. *Social Science Information, 16*, 645–668.

Bourdieu, P. (1991). *Language and symbolic power* (G. Raymond & M. Adamson, Trans.). Cambridge, MA: Harvard University Press.

Chang, J. (2005). *Can't stop, won't stop: A history of the hip-hop generation*. New York, NY: St. Martin's Press.

Denzin, N. (2003). *Performance ethnography: Critical pedagogy and the politics of culture*. Thousand Oaks, CA: SAGE.

Dixson, A., & Rousseau, C. (Eds.). (2006). *Critical race theory in education: All God's children got a song*. New York, NY: Routledge,

Fanon, F. (1967). *Black skin white Mask*. New York, NY: Grove Weidenfeld.

Freire, P. (1993). *Pedagogy of the oppressed*. New York, NY: Continuum.

Hall, S. (1996). Introduction: Who needs "Identity"? In S. Hall & P. du Gay (Eds.) *Questions of Cultural Identity* (pp. 1–21). London, England: SAGE.

Heller, M. (2006). *Linguistic minorities and modernity: A sociolinguistic ethnography*. New York, NY: Continuum.

Ibrahim, A. (2000). "Whassup Homeboy?" Black/popular culture and the politics of "Curriculum Studies": Devising an anti-racism perspective. In G. J. Dei & A. Calliste (Eds.), *Power, knowledge and anti-racism education* (pp. 57–72). Halifax, Canada: Fernwood.

Ibrahim, A. (2003). May 16, 1999: The story of the "dark man." *Inquiry: Critical Thinking Across the Discipline, 21*(3), 23–26.

Ibrahim, A. (2004). Operating under erasure: ~~Hip-hop~~ and the pedagogy of affect(ive). *Journal of Curriculum Theorizing, 20*(1), 113–133.

Ibrahim, A. (2006). Rethinking displacement, language, and culture shock: Towards a pedagogy of cultural translation and negotiation. In N. Amin & G. Dei (Eds.), *The poetics of anti-racism* (pp. 33–45). Halifax, Canada: Fernwood Books.

Ibrahim, A. (2011). When life is off da hook: Hip-hop identity and identification, BESL, and the pedagogy of pleasure. In C. Higgins (Ed.), *Negotiating the self in another language: Identity formation in a globalized world* (pp. 221–238). Berlin, Germany: Mouton de Gruyter.

Ibrahim, A. (2014). *The rhizome of Blackness: A critical ethnography of hip-hop culture, language, identity, and the politics of becoming*. New York, NY: Peter Lang.

Ibrahim, A. (2016). "Who Owns My Language?" African Canadian youth, post-coloniality and the Yymbolic violence of language in a French-language high school in Ontario. In A. Ibrahim & A. Abdi (Eds.), *The education of African Canadian Children: Critical perspectives* (pp. 145–163). Montreal, Canada: McGill-Queen's University Press.

Ng-A-Fook, N., Ibrahim, A., & Reis, G. (2016). *Provoking curriculum studies: Strong poetry and the arts of the possible in education*. New York, NY: Routledge.

Norton, B., & Toohey, K. (2004). *Critical pedagogies and language learning*. Cambridge, England: Cambridge University Press.

Ortner, S. (2006). *Anthropology and social theory: Culture, power, and the acting subject*. Duke, NC: Duke University Press.

Peirce, N. (1995). Social identity, investment, and language learning. *TESOL Quarterly, 29*(1) 9–31.

Philip, M. N. (1991). *Harriet's daughter*. Toronto, ON: The Women's Press.

Morgan, B. (1998). *The ESL classroom: Teaching, critical practice, and community development*. Toronto, ON: University of Toronto Press.

Rabinow, P. [Foucault, M.]. (1984). *The Foucault reader*. New York, NY: Pantheon Books.

Rose, T. (1991). "Fear of a Black Planet": Rap music and Black cultural politics in the 1990. *Journal of Negro Education, 60*(3), 276–290.

Shaw-Taylor, Y., & Tuch, S. (Eds.). (2007). *The other African Americans: Contemporary African and Caribbean immigrants in the United States*. Lanham, MD: Rowman & Littlefield Simon.

Simon R. I., & Dippo, D. (1986). On critical ethnography work. *Anthropology & Education Quarterly, 17*, 195–202.

Simmons, M. (2016). Diaspora, citizenry, becoming human, and the education of African Canadian youth. In A. Ibrahim & A. Abdi (Eds.), *The education of African Canadian children: Critical perspectives* (pp. 58–72). Montreal, Canada: McGill-Queen's University Press.

Simon, R., & Dippo, D. (1986). On critical ethnography work. *Anthropology and Education Quarterly 17*, 195–202.

Smitherman, G. (2000). *Black talk: Words and phrases from the hood to the amen corner*. Boston, MA: Houghton Mifflin.

Steinberg, S. (2014). Redefining the notion of youth: Contextualizing the possible for transformative youth leadership. In A. Ibrahim & S. Steinberg (Eds.), *Critical youth studies reader* (pp. 426–433). New York, NY: Peter Lang.

Toohey, K. (2000). *Learning English at school: Identity, social relations and classroom practice*. Clevedon, England: Multilingual Matters.

CHAPTER 8

THE ONTOLOGICAL PROBLEM OF CONTEMPORARY U.S. EDUCATION

A Non-linear, Sensuous Critique

Walter S. Gershon
Kent State University

A kindergarten teacher who is pursuing her master's in education at a large state university receives a reading assignment in a text designed for graduate students and remarks, "I don't get this and I shouldn't have to read it, I'm just a kindergarten teacher."

A public middle school (Grades 6–8) makes a policy decision to lock the doors to the bathrooms during students' 5-minute passing periods to ensure that students are on time to class. They are unlocked during nutritional break and lunch and girls are permitted to keep a spare change of clothes in the nurses' office. School colors for the mandatory dress code are beige pants/skirts and blue shirts/tops.

Sensuous Curriculum:
Politics and the Senses in Education, pp. 135–156

> *A Latino fourth grader* is moving his body rhythmically while he does his math assignment. His teacher, who is also Latino and grew up in the same neighborhood as the student, negatively sanctions the student stating that he "needs to stop messing around and get back to work." Already finished with his assignment (he had nine of ten answers correct), he stops moving and makes an effort not to move for the next 8 minutes while his peers finish their work.

These are but three examples of the material consequences for the ontological problem that is contemporary education in the United States. This is not simply a case of sublimating ways of being for ways of knowing, although such sublimation is certainly often the case in American educational theory and practice. Nor is this only a call for a return to considering a person not solely in terms of her cognition in educational interactions such as teaching and learning, while this is also certainly a point of no small importance. Put bluntly, a lack of attention and action to processes of educational ontology has created an orientation towards curriculum, pedagogy, and studenting that is harmful for all students and continues a tradition of unequal educational opportunities in a systematic and consistent manner (cf. Cooper, 1892; Brown & Brown, 2010; Valenzuela, 2005; Watkins, 2011; Winfield, 2007; Woodson, 1933). Although such an argument may seem like hyperbole, as I articulate here, this may in fact be an understatement.

This argument is predicated on an understanding that processes of making sense lie at the heart of educational interactions of teaching and learning are processes of sensation and signification (Gershon, 2011, 2013, 2017a). Furthermore, without sensation there can be no signification (cf. Dewey, 1929; Howes, 2003; Stoller, 1997; Woodson, 1933). As a result, how one "is"—one's continually emergent, socioculturally and historically contextualized, complexly intermediated ways of being—is a strong determinant not only one's for ways of knowing but also the ideas and ideals that count as knowledge (e.g., Caponi, 1999; Hemmings, 2006; Mills, 1998; Sedgewick, 2003). It is these layered understandings that form what is ordinarily sensible, the everyday ways people make sense.

Part of the difficulty of this argument is that it is largely theoretical on one hand, and, other the other, a lack of attention to what I call ontogenic (following Massumi, 2002, who speaks of the ontogenetic), the fluid state of emergent ontology, is so pervasive as to appear normal. Speaking to this concern therefore requires tacking back and forth between the theoretical and the material as well as between very localized exemplars and the broader contexts in which those instances are situated.

This approach is in many ways parallel to how Brian Massumi (2002) articulates the relations between "movement, affect and sensation" and the ways in which Anna Lowenhaupt Tsing (2005) charts local and global frictions in her strong ethnography on the often-negative consequences of globalization. In different ways towards occasionally different ends, both Tsing and Massumi insist on the fluidity of ideas, ideals, and processes as well as the inseparability between making sense, sensation, signification, and power.

This kind of fluidity also engenders a slightly different approach to narrative and explication. Part of what makes such an argument difficult lies in the fact that English is in many ways not linguistically structured to attend to the ontological. The Japanese word 雰囲気 (pronounced foo-eehn-key) is but one example. While it is usually translated in English as "atmosphere" or "mood" the character's mean "atmosphere-enclosed[space]-spirit/way." When one describes a space as 雰囲気, one means that the atmosphere of a space resonates with one's spirit or way of being; not quite the same as when one walks into a restaurant and says that it has a good atmosphere or the mood is right, although this is often how 雰囲気 is translated into English.

As scholars in affect theory, sensory studies, and others have noted, another key difficulty is that Western constructions of meaning tend to focus their attention to ideas as static and to foreground, often in rather colonial ways and an othering manner, the centrality of signification over all other ways of knowing (Caponi, 1999; Classen, 1993; Clough& Halley, 2007; Geurts, 2002; Gregg & Seigworth, 2011; Howes, 2009; Stoller, 1997). In education, this can be seen in examples such as the uses and abuses of written language, IQ tests and the propagation of eugenic ideologies, and the construction of difference as deficit both in and out of schools (e.g., Gershon, 2012; Pennington, 2005; Valencia, 2010; Watkins, 2011; Winfield, 2007).

What is perhaps of most significance for the argument in this article are connections between ethics, social justice, and the ontogenic. Similarly, constructions of the "is-ness" of educational ideas and ideals, institutions, people, interactions and ecologies deeply impact both the possibilities for how they "be" and the ways in which their "be-ing" is perceived.

As but one concrete example, students are most often "in trouble" in daily classroom interactions not for how they think or learn but instead for who they *are* and how they *be* (Gershon, 2012, 2017b). Academically, students are most often in trouble for falsely representing work as theirs (cheating/plaigiarism) or not providing an answer closely enough to the one their teacher prescribed (an ontological problem of its own for what if the student is also correct but not in the manner her teacher anticipated?). Socially, however, students are in trouble for a whole host of reasons related to their is-ness. This plays out not only in ways where differences in students' social, cultural, racial, economic, gender, sexual preference, linguistic, age, perceived able-body-ness but also in the ordinarily sensible.

For example, I once witnessed the following series of events. The only African American girl in a fifth grade class was asked to put her head down after completing a task designed as part of a study in a university computer lab. First one of the research assistants asked her to pick her head up and do her work; then another assistant made the same request. When the student replied okay to each request then again put her head down, the teaching assistant who traveled with the class to the university lab came up and told the student in a stern, raised voice that she was being defiant. At this, the student, to her surprising credit, neither cried nor yelled back but instead stated that she had been asked to stay at her seat when she finished answering the 10 questions on the screen. She had, so she was quietly waiting as requested. The student not only was the first to finish but also got 9 out of 10 of the prompts correct.

No one apologized to her. Regardless of whether it was her Blackness, her girl-ness, her speed, her quietly respectful non-response to adults' lack of understanding, or, most likely, some combination of the above that got her in trouble, it was nonetheless her is-ness rather than her thinking for which she was negatively sanctioned.

As noted above, such an attention to race and ontology has a long history in relation to schooling in the United States (e.g. Cooper, 1892; DuBois, 1903; Watkins, 2001; Woodson, 1933). In particular, scholars such as Anna Julia Cooper, Mary Jane McLeod Bethnune, Angela Y. Davis, Charlotte Forten, bell hooks, and other women of color have noted the added often-negative consequences when gender further complicates the intersection of race, ontology and school. These understandings of ontological differences as deficits can also be seen throughout a wide range of educational literature, in the work of such scholars as Ray R. Rist (e.g., 1973), Beverly Gordon (e.g., 1993), Pauline Lipman (1998), and Lisa Delpit (2006, 2013).

This scholarship is significant and the fact that the work of Bethune, Cooper, DuBois, McLoed, Woodson, and others are still not foundational readings in many teacher education programs is a null curriculum that needs to be addressed in a direct and immediate fashion. Similar constructions of difference as deficit (Valencia, 1997) in ways of being can be seen, for example, in First Nations/Native American—White tensions in schooling (e.g., Donald, 2009; Grande, 2004; Ng-A-Fook, 2007). Furthermore, as Mills (1998) strongly argues, the ontological is indeed social and the racial is often overlooked in questions of philosophy in general and of ontology in specific (also Gershon, 2017b; Roelofs, 2009).

However, my point here is not only that there is a long history of systematically casting people's of color ways of being as something other than normal with a similarly long history of negative, material results for children, youth, young adults, and teachers in schools. It is my argument that a systematic and continuing lack of attention to what it means to "be" one's self and the myriad ways a person can make sense in school has negative concrete, material consequences. These consequences impact *all* students' and teachers' lives and trajectories both in and out of school. It is a position that takes at its core that schooling in the United States negatively impacts all children and, simultaneously, even further marginalizes non-dominant groups' and individuals' ontologies. In sum, I contend that contemporary education in the United States has an ontological problem that is met with epistemological justifications, rather than an epistemological problem that can be recognized in its ontological manifestations.

Finally, this piece addresses not only the ontological but also the ontogenic. In this way, the arguments here also comment on what Schwab called the "curriculum-in-action," the enacted curriculum. For it is in the everyday emergent moments of being and knowing that one "is" and can "be." In light of what seems to be a recent dearth of discussions that pertain to the enacted curriculum—often in favor of considerations of hidden and null curricula and, more recently, a trend that returns to questions of formal curriculum in response to ever-increasing layers of standardized assessment and accompanying curricula—this piece can also be understood as a call for a more explicit returning of attention to the enacted curriculum (e.g., Gershon, 2017b).

Here, I have adopted a fluid, somewhat experimental manner that moves not only back and forth in scale (Helfenbein, 2009) but also in style, an approach that draws from possibilities created by scholars such as Patti Lather and Chris Smithies' (1997) *Troubling the Angels: Women Living with HIV/AIDS*, Alma Gottlieb and Philip Graham's (2012) *Braided Worlds*, Ruth Behar's (199) *The Vulnerable Observer: Anthropology that Breaks Your Heart*, and, particularly, Kathleen Stewart's (2007) *Ordinary Affects*. Aspects of this work also address points I have raised in other contexts towards different ends and with different trajectories (Gerhson, 2012, 2013, 2017b). It is an intentionally woven work with a philosophical warp and a narrative weft, entwined in the effort to create a theoretical piece of material value.

In this case, my purpose is to draw attention to the ways in which the ontological is simultaneously a seminal part of everyday experiences yet is markedly and consistently absent, if not purposefully targeted for removal, in many central aspects of contemporary education in the United States. As with the style of the creatively narrative works that inform this article, I have done so in order to articulate the extraordinary nature of the ordinarily sensible, everyday acts of sensation and signification, of making sense. Rather than a linear and sequential directionality towards specific resolution, this piece is intentionally performative, seeking to articulate resonances between ideas and their material consequences in a somewhat paradoxical fashion, writing so that the ordinarily consonant becomes dissonant in a manner that renders the familiar strange and the strange again familiar.

INTERRUPTING EPISTEMOLOGY: THREE CONSTRUCTIONS OF KNOWING

Following its Western and Eurocentric roots, it is often the case that scholarship in and about American education explicitly or implicitly works from an understanding that one must know something in order to name that thing. Such an understanding is evident from the ways in which teachers are taught to deliver curricula to the manner in which students are to express the knowledge they are to have learned. Interrupting such a linear construction of knowing-to-naming are three maxims and their expressions in everyday moments of schooling.

1. One can know something one cannot name
2. One can name something that one cannot fully describe
3. One can name something one does not know

A student walks over to his friend and gently bumps his shoulder into his friend's, and immediately his friend's body language changes—shoulders that were slumped straighten, arms relax, as he turns to smile. Two girls sit across from each other day after day eating lunch together in the cafeteria then, suddenly, one day, they both realize at the same time that they were right about one another and can quietly relax in their mutual crush. One can know something that one cannot name.

Teachable moments. An educator intuitively understands when a teachable moment has arrived and orients her affective attention to her role as teacher in order to be as alert for such moments as possible. Like an epiphany, she can recognize that moment when it arrives and may well be able to trace a series of events (Massumi, 2011) for the sensation, interaction, or idea that served as its trigger. However, although both events have names that are commonly used and are experiences that are explicitly sought by educators (writ large), both teachable moments and epiphanies in many ways defy definitive explanation. One can talk about the experience but the experience of the event is a kind of embodied, affectively liminal moment that tends to be very difficult to name. One can name something one cannot fully describe.

In every secondary math class there are students who are excellent at procedure. Their papers start with a mathematical problem, move through each step exactly as they have been shown, and arrive at the correct answers. They matriculate through each grade and receive high scores in math, often in ways that allow them to pass out of basic math in college. However, these students cannot explain the ideas behind the procedures in which they are engaged. Instead, they have learned to count on the righteousness of the procedure, a "virtue" that is privileged to the point that, like all forms of privilege, they are free not to notice that they might not understand the underlying mathematical concept. Additionally, the privileging of correct procedures is such that others such as teachers and peers similarly don't notice their lack of understanding.

Here the assumption is that a correctness of procedure is an indicator of the comprehension of an idea or ideas. The difficulty with this assumption is that it conflates two separate aspects of learning, procedural correctness with comprehension. However, it is the case that (a) one can complete a procedure without knowing the concept a procedure demonstrates or that (b) one can understand a concept yet not be able to demonstrate that knowledge in a way that can be registered as procedurally correct. One can name something one does not know.

That one can know things one cannot name, have important educational experiences that one cannot describe, and document educational procedures one does not know raises important questions about what counts as education in this historical moment. As significantly, it questions the ways in which students, teachers, and schools are currently adjudicated as educated and/or educative.

A SCHOOL IS BOT A PERSON

In the United States, a business is a person. A corporation is similarly a person and also accorded many of the same rights as a person. For, as the rationale goes, a business is formed by groups of people. The economy is often conceptualized in terms of the market, singular, and is also anthropomorphized. It is not just whether the market is up or down, directionalities in trading that are often also equated with emotions, but it is also provided with other adjectives that describe how this construction feels. Its affect impacts people just as people impact the market. Additionally, money is speech. A person can now spend it with the same fluidity as they would talk about an idea. The more money a person has, the greater their voice. This also means that, in spite of the fact that businesses of all sizes are comprised of people with a variety of roles, incomes, and other resources, a business is often considered as a singularity and that singularity tends to be granted the same emotions and rights as a person. In this way, the more money a corporation, business, group of individuals, or individual has, the greater their voice.

A public school is not a person. It is not anthropomorphized like a business, the market, the economy, Congress, or the (Supreme) Court. This raises some important questions about the people in schools. For example, why are children occasionally referred to as "our most precious resource," a move that equates a human being with their economic worth, yet the place that provides for the growth of that resource not given the same status as money or business? One answer is that it is an ontological absence that contributes to a narrowing of epistemological possibilities.

A HELPING PROFESSION VERSUS A SERVICE INDUSTRY

Contemporary P–12 education in the United States is now largely a process of accounting. Students, teachers, schools and school districts are measured by students' successes on standardized assessments. Standardized curricula designed to ensure that students have a broad set of understandings have come to function as correct answers on selected response questions.

School districts buy textbooks from publishing houses that have worked hard to create curricula that provide the necessary information for students to score well on their standardized assessments, texts that vary according to each state's annual assessment needs. In some cases, larger school districts purchase textbooks with an understanding that they will increase students' test scores on annual assessments, agreements that entail a provision that teachers deliver the content according to the textbook's design. Increasingly, publishing houses are also providing not only textbooks but also the standardize assessments for entire states.

Teachers at all levels are provided access to coaches in the key areas of literacy and mathematics whose job it is to ensure that teachers are teaching the textbooks in the prescribed manner and to further help teachers and their students arrive at the understandings as provided in the textbooks. Students' grades as well as teachers' pay and ability to keep their jobs have been tied to students' test scores. A teacher's job has in many ways become the ability to successfully deliver the correct answers in a way that students can retain so that they score well on their tests; scores that carry the double weight of not only determining multiple layers of success but are also strong determinants in students' placement for classes in the following academic year.

In colleges and universities, state policies increasingly call for an accounting of professors' success according to their future teachers' success as a teacher, successes that are in turn measured by their future students' test scores on their annual standardized assessments—professors' current success measured by future teachers' future students' scores. Professors are evaluated according to their scores on students' evaluations, scores that are in many cases also tied to tenure and promotion, regardless of students' comfort with the topics of the course or factors such as whether or not a course is a mandatory part of a sequence or a course chosen by the student because of her interest.

Teachers at all levels are focused on best practices. There are, however, three central concerns with the notion that any one practice might be best. First, it carries universalist assumptions that human beings' myriad differences might all be approached with a singular set of understandings about how they best conceptualize and retain ideas, ideals and processes. Second, similar to Kliebard's (2004) critique of Ralph Tyler's use of teaching as measurable goals and objectives and Bill Readings's (1996) critique of excellence at the university, what is "best" is often determined by a group of experts who have a vested capital (both sociocultural and economic) interest in schooling and school. What is a best practice is often a resonance between those with voice and agency to make decisions about what the art of teaching means and the ideas, as well as the individuals who generated the concepts that those in power wish to deliver to students. Third, placing the previous two understandings along side one another, best practices tend to come from the business world where the goal is to create particular products through replicable processes in order to increase revenue. However, people learn in a multitude of manners and, as most teachers, parents, and other educators already understand, not necessarily according to a particular timetable. When combined, best practices create a context in which one educational process or tool is applied universally regardless of context. Only for the intellectual elite is best practices not best practices, in medical, law, and doctoral programs for example.

The move here seems to be away from education as a process for affective, social, and intellectual growth, instead firmly locating education as a content delivery system for formal curricular product. As such, rather than a helping profession geared towards a person's development, education has become a service industry, closer to delivering desired goods than considering possibilities. Students, particularly at the university level, have come to be conceptualized more like customers whose educational expectations need to be satisfied rather than helped like doctors, provided knowledge that might not be familiar or comfortable to the person who receives it but vital nonetheless. This has in many ways turned teaching into a service industry and away from its roots as a helping profession. Concretely, as a sign in a local high school meeting room (see Figure 8.1 on next page) clearly states:

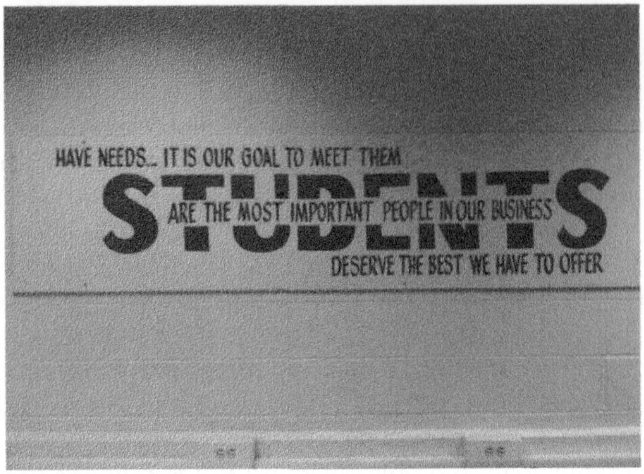
HAVE NEEDS... IT IS OUR GOAL TO MEET THEM
STUDENTS
ARE THE MOST IMPORTANT PEOPLE IN OUR BUSINESS
DESERVE THE BEST WE HAVE TO OFFER

Figure 8.1.

TEACHING AND LEARNING

Teachers teach and learners learn. Although there is a good deal of overlap between these interactions and roles, strong teaching does not necessarily elicit learning and one can learn well in spite of poor teaching. Where all teachers' interactions can be understood as teaching regardless of their actual educational value, students' interactions are not all considered to be learning. In general, it is teachers, not students, who determine whether or not students are learning, choices that can be made without asking students what they might have learned. Similarly, as noted above, a P–12 teacher's success in the U.S. is often determined by students' scores on annual assessments and without asking students either what they have learned or what students think of their teachers' teaching.

In order to create a space where teachers' successes can be determined by students' scores and teachers' can determine student success without engaging students requires a conflation of experiences and interactions of teaching and learning. One must blur the lines between these two so that teaching is equated with learning to create the following axiom: strong teaching necessarily begets strong learning. The difficulty with this construction of the relationship between teaching and learning, as noted above, is that teachers can teach very well and students might not learn and that teachers can teach poorly and students can learn in spite of a teacher's teaching. Just ask the third grade teacher whose job it is each year to introduce the next group of students to long division.

THE PARADOXICAL PERILS OF A LESSON PLAN

The difficulty of a lesson plan lies in a paradox for new teachers (and often remains throughout a teacher's career). On one hand, they are new to teaching and need some way to articulate what it is they plan to teach as well as the kinds of interactions through which they intend to engender students' learning. On the other, newness and other factors such as constant surveillance by their cooperating teacher during their student teaching period can lead beginning teachers to overly adhere to their lesson plan, occasionally in spite of whether or not students are either interested or learning.

Further, the very real pressures new and experienced teachers alike now face to have their students score well on standardized assessments creates a context in which an annual curriculum map or the teacher's edition of a textbook serve not as a guide but as a script. The purpose, the argument runs, is to ensure that students have the necessary information to be successful as judged by their scores on state mandated, federally encouraged standardized assessments. And those assessments do matter for they have become one of the central sorting mechanisms for students' successes and failures in school (see, for example, Varenne & McDermott, 1998 on the binary of school success and failures and McNeil, 2000 as well as Valli, Croninger, Chambliss, Graeber & Buese, 2008 and Taubman, 2009, on the impact of standardized assessments on classrooms). Such pressures often also contribute to a lack of attention to the affective connections between classroom actors (most of students and teachers) and an increased focus on narrowing epsitemologies and correct answers (for a critique of "correct" in complexity sciences, see Davis & Sumara, 2006, pp. 38–42)

Additionally, many school districts have also adopted a policy of quarterly internal assessments given to gauge students' learning during the year in order to better evaluate students' progress so that they might receive either more support to be potentially successful on their next standardized assessment. Students are also often sorted and resorted into relatively homogenous groups according to these internal assessments so that they might better receive the attention they need to progress towards the goal of being on grade level as determined by their annual federal and state mandated assessments.

In order that students receive the requisite content prior to their annual assessment each spring, and on their quarterly district-produced assessments for those that have them, it is often necessary for teachers to follow the curriculum map produced at the beginning of the academic year before the students arrive. This raises an important question. If lesson and unit plans must be followed in order that students might be successful on their assessments, and daily lessons move forward accordingly regardless of students' comprehension so that the prescribed content is covered, why is there any need for students?

ENGLISH LANGUAGE LEARNER

Jorge was a fifth grader in an elementary school in one of the barrios of the San Fernando Valley just north and east of Los Angeles. Students who attended the school were majority Latin@ and Mexican@. Jorge is a first generation American who was also a strong student and kind person, always willing to help a peer who might not have understood something he did and inclusive on the yard in whatever game he was playing. Jorge also had a tendency to ask either insightful questions or the kinds of questions that others were also wondering but were less comfortable asking, the sort of questions where the teacher was less clear than he had thought and had moved on as if everything were copasetic.

Jorge was his family's translator. He translated at his and his younger two siblings' parent-teacher conferences, at all of his family members' doctors appointments, and was the person who took English calls at his house regardless of their content.

Jorge was also unable to remove his distinction as what was then called an ELL, an English language learner. Granted, he was a level 5 ELL, the highest category possible while still retaining the designation, but an ELL nonetheless. His inability to shake this possibility had little to do with his written, spoken or read English. Instead, it was a combination of the fact that his parents had written on a mandatory reporting paper that they spoke Spanish in their house and at the changing nature of the final assessment to drop his ELL status. (In contrast many of the immigrant Armenian families whose students had the cultural capital to know to write that their home language was English as to avoid an issue like this one for their children.) Two years after leaving the school to pursue his graduate studies full time at a university for which the drive time in the Southern California traffic prevented his continuing to work at the elementary school, the teacher heard that Jorge was no longer ELL from one of his previous colleagues who was also Jorge's neighbor. Unfortunately, she noted, the change in designation might not be in time to get him into the honors English classes comparable to the books he was reading at the time.

LITERACIES

The difficulty with literacy and literacies is not in the importance of being literate. Nor is the problem with the notion that there are multiple literacies or that such pluralities can be viewed through critical lenses and sociocultural/socioeconomic/sociolinguistic contexts. At this moment, the problems with literacies seem to be an ahistoriocity coupled with an overreach. Historically, literacy was born of illiteracy, a positive possibility in the face of its negative parent (Janks, 2007). This, in turn, creates a context in which everything that might be called a literacy must necessarily have people who are illiterate. Literacy also has a history of being a tool for colonization (Pennington, 2005) and for domination in education (Winfield, 2007).

Furthermore, less like the arts and humanities, literacy has a history if not a practice of being able to be parsed into discreetly measurable skills. Again, the problem lies not in that such skills can be measured or that they are discreet for literacies such as critical media literacy, the skills through which one decontextualizes and otherwise unpacks messages and media, are central to interrupting unequal power structures. However, it is not a critical language art with its history in the humanities and tinges of the aesthetically political and affectively liminal that has become *de rigeur*, but is instead the frame and lens of literacy with its history of identifying the practically and socioculturally illiterate that has become the model as can be seen throughout the "Common Core Standards."

Additionally, critically reading interactions as texts has deep advantages in that it can create snapshots out of movements and critique those moments that would ordinarily pass us by. The ability to still or distill ideas, ideals, interactions, ecologies, or processes as textual representations, allows them to be deconstructed or otherwise critically considered in ways that would likely not be possible without their stillness. Along similar lines, as Howes (2003) notes, the textual can provide distance so that the reader can less readily mistake the recording for the completeness of an event as might happen with representation via video. However, a text is not a sound, a smell, a taste or an experience; visual metaphors are as constraining as they are enabling and are often the tools of the literate used to manipulate those they consider less so.

Then there is the overreach. A literacy is not an experience (Dewey, 1929, 1998/1934). A person's way of being is not a literacy, even those that are critical and contextually aware, are often ways of knowing that tend to privilege signification over sensation. How one knows is important in as much as it relates to how one "is." Is how one feels upon hearing one's child cry for the first time a literacy? Is the feeling of being pushed on the playground because of the color of one's skin a literacy? Is the taste of honey or the feeling of love a literacy?

BETA TESTING ON STUDENTS

Every so often a new set of policy initiatives strongly informs how teachers, students, schools, and by a very slight inference, communities are adjudicated and otherwise understood. Although the very public measurement of schools against each other by a system of scoring ending in excellence at first glance appears to be new, there is a long history of dividing American students and their communities into successes and failures through schooling (e.g., McDermott & Aron, 1978; Varenne & McDermott, 1998).

Publishing houses and other content delivery systems (e.g. developers of "hands on" science kits) are continually updating and developing new curricula, often in the form of textbooks, teacher's guides, student workbooks, and so forth. The tone and tenor of recent changes of this kind are in many ways radically different in qualitative ways that have significant material consequences for students, teachers, schools and districts (e.g., Alonso, Anderson, Su, & Theoharis, 2009; Anderson, 2009; Gershon, 2017b; Valli, Croninger, Chambliss, Graeber, & Buese, 2008).

However, there is a continuing tradition in such changes. As such, educational policies and curriculum are developed, they are then sold to districts and, less frequently, to schools. With increasing developments in technology, curricula tend to be delivered with greater rapidity. Nevertheless, the following practice is relatively consistent. Most often, a first set of focused delivery provided to test the ways a given text or system of text(book)s functions when put into daily practice in schools and then again when new curricula are again sold to more districts, books, terms, ideas, and ideals that are tweaked and re-tweaked until they reach their desired results. In the language of technology (textbooks) and commerce (publishing houses), curricula are beta tested on children.

Additionally, these textbooks are geared towards students' passing their annual standardized assessments and tweaked every couple of years in light of both changes on those assessments and students' success at passing them. It is also increasingly the case that the same publishing house is at once providing the curricula students are to learn and the standardized assessments through which they are measured. This adjusting curricula to better fit the assessments designed and designing assessments to better fit the curricula designed is a process that produces a well-designed closed set of beta testing in which both curricula and assessment are continually tested and retested on students. Unlike the children who have only one shot at either curriculum or assessment and are judged accordingly before moving on, the curricula and assessments are in a seemingly endless feedback loop of adjustment that benefits from students' participation as subjects in these beta tests regardless of their success or failure. It is a system that benefits at the expense of children regardless of the benefits they receive as a result of their participation.

A GIRL, AN OWL, AND AN ASSESSMENT

A kindergartener takes an assessment with her peers. The assessment finds that she is well below grade level in the areas of listening and speaking. Concerned, her parents go to meet the reading specialist in charge of the assessments. When asked to see the assessment the parents note that their daughter was marked down for the following two corrections:

1. Instead of exactly repeating, "If the boy touches the hot stove he might get burned," their daughter had stated, "If the boy touches the hot stove, he *will* get burned."
2. Their daughter moved an adverbial clause from the beginning to the middle of a phrase, a second grade standard.

When the parents objected to these two issues on the grounds that the first was what she and most young children have been taught, hot stoves tend to burn and should not be touched, and that the second was a more advanced use of language, the reading specialist replied that although that might be the case, those were not the correct answers. The parents then saw that there was a space for the specialist to write in any notes associated with the assessment, that their daughter did not have any issues with listening and/or or speaking or that she had clearly understood both the prompt and its implications, for example. The reading specialist refused on the grounds that doing so would be against the rules of the assessment and, in an endless feedback loop of paradoxical irony, only a specialist could do so.

Because the parents were making no headway with the specialist who claimed only a specialist could make notes on an assessment, the principal was called in to the meeting. The principal quickly understood the parents' concern and facilitated that a note be added by the specialist in her role as the professional who had the power to do so and had their daughter retake the assessment with him.

When meeting with the principal later, he shared a story about their daughter taking a similar assessment with a different specialist given to all kindergarteners in the state. As part of the assessment, their daughter was asked to draw a person. The person giving the test marked her drawing as incorrect. The principal, who was also in the room helping to give the assessment, happened to see this assessment and the scorer's mark. He asked their daughter what she had drawn.

An owl, she replied.

But you were supposed to draw a person, the principal responded, would you do that please?

Their daughter then added a head and some legs to her drawing and said, There, it's an owl person.

The response cracked the principal up and he marked her drawing as correct, for she had not only fulfilled the purpose of the exercise (she could demonstrate she knew the different body parts of a person and where they might go) but she had also found a creative solution through critical reflection of her problem—that she wanted to draw an owl, was more comfortable drawing an owl than a person, but was told she had to draw a person.

The assessments followed similar patterns and the child in both cases was the same person. The difference was in the adults' ways of being, approaches to the world that inhibited or enabled their understanding of their role as educator. That testing is designed to negatively mark imagination, creativity, and critical inquiry in children so young also speaks to the narrowness of epistemological possibilities as the result of an inattention to the ontogenic.

MOVEMENT IN RELATION

Who one is determines how and what one knows ways of being so ordinary that they feel natural in spite of their multiple layers of mediation. Yet how one is affects not only learning but also movement in relation to others, ecologies, ideas, ideals, and other processes.

MAKING SENSE OF CONTEMPORARY EDUCATIONAL WAYS OF BEING AND KNOWING

In addition to the ways in which U.S. education has been conceptualized in the field of curriculum studies (e.g., Kliebard, 2004; Schubert, 1985), education can also be understood as tensions between three constructions regarding the purpose of education: education for a strong citizenry, education for a strong economy or workforce, and education for knowledge's sake. However, there is little room in contemporary standards-based assessment-driven education for discussions of citizenship education or social studies in general (cf. Wills, 2006). The national discussion for the need to prepare future generations of workers in science, technology, engineering, and mathematics is a strong indicator that schools are not producing the kinds of workers that business and industry project they will need. Additionally, given the ways in which school knowledge and ways of being in "doing school" has become most associated with what Mehan (1979) called "known information questions"—questions to which there is a single correct answer that is already known rather than open ended inquiry—it would appear that this particular way of doing school is not geared towards education for a more broad and deep set of knowledge.

This does not mean that contemporary schooling is not successful for it is most certainly moving ever-resolutely forward. A central question then becomes, what kind of education is contemporary American schooling working towards, what are students being prepared to do? What knowledge is considered to be worthy of knowing?

One possible answer to this question is to treat the educational system anthropomorphically, the system as a person. A central goal for all species is self-perpetuation. Through this lens, it would appear as though schools are successfully continuing practices of ensuring that students are divided according to visible sociocultural makers like race and gender and less visible markers like class, language, gender identity and expression, and sexual orientation. It would also seem as though that what most public school students might be best prepared for when they graduate high school is not college, particularly to hear professors who teach undergraduates in state schools talk, nor the workforce, to hear both small and big business leaders talk. What public school students are perhaps best prepared for is to be future public school teachers who would then use their particularized skill sets to begin training the next generation of future teachers. It is the iteratively recursive processes of a closed, self-perpetuating system, a Mobius strip endlessly cycling around itself rather than an act of intellectual fission in which the process is a catalyst for myriad possibilities.

SOCIAL JUSTICE IS

One trick of social justice is that it is. It is more in the doing and in one's ways of being than in the ideas that frame those possibilities. For a person can think she is being just when she is just being fair or one can intellectually conflate the ideas of justice with acting justly. This is also a central concern with additive constructions of social justice on one hand and universalist constructions of social justice on the other. Both assume that social justice is ideas or processes that can be either mapped onto existing structures and that one person's justice is similar in kind to another's. This is not the case (Ayers, Quinn, & Stovall, 2008; Tsing, 2005, 2015). Social justice is in the being and the doing, it is a feedback loop of the ontogenic that engenders epistemologies of hope.

EDUCATION AS THE CONSTRUCTION OF THE ORDINARILY SENSIBLE

Education is about making sense, the myriad processes and interactions of sensation and signification. Because learning, both in and out of formal (institutional) contexts like schools, tends to reside in people's daily experiences, what is sensible is the multitude of ordinary commonplace ways that ideas, ideals, bodies, experiences, ecologies, animals, and objects make sense to a given person. As described above, how one makes sense at any given moment of any given experience is contextualized by their construction of previous moments of sense making and projects into the future as a set of conditions and possibilities for ways that person might make sense in the future. The point here is not that what is ordinarily sensible is not extraordinary but that the extraordinary becomes ordinary once one believes that they have made sense of sensations and significations.

From this perspective, education is a process of making previously extraordinary things ordinarily sensible. Therefore, because the ordinarily sensible is ontogenic as much as it is epistemogenic, the ontological is as central to education as the epistemological. Furthermore, if how one is strongly determines both how and what one knows, then ignoring the ontogenic and considering the epistemogenic only in its static form of epistemology is not only bad educational practice but also willfully harmful to all students and learning in general and to particularly damaging to traditionally marginalized students and their learning in specific.

EVERYTHING OLD IS NEW AGAIN (AGAIN)

Ontology has always been central to teaching and learning. How one is indeed shapes how one knows, the ontogenic flowing into the epistemogenic in a never-ending, iteratively recursive feedback loop of gaining and transmitting information. It has, however, often been bracketed or seen as a vehicle for ways of knowing, a lingering Hegelianism with a Cartesian twist. Nevertheless, Anna Julia Cooper, W.E.B. Dubois, John Dewey, Sojourner Truth, George Counts, Maxine Greene, Ted T. Aoki, and countless others have over and again documented the importance of ways of being to educational processes like teaching and learning.

I IS, I BE, I AM

A group five of alternative high school students are sitting in a row at the front of a classroom. Filling the rest of the classroom are approximately 45 master's in teaching students who are in an intensive one-year program to simultaneously receive a master's in education and a teaching credential. The alternative high school students have been placed in the somewhat uncomfortable position of being asked by a local administrator to serve on a panel, the purpose of which is to share with these future high school teachers the following: (a) the kinds of interactions and choices they made that caused them to be identified as at-risk enough to be part of the district's alternative program and (b) how the alternative school differs from the afternoons they spend at the non-alternative "regular" high school they all attend. Having shared their experiences, the high school students are now taking questions from the preservice teachers who are their audience. After a few questions, the following exchange occurs:

Preservice Teacher Question:	What does a comfortable school environment consist of?
Alternative School Student Answer:	Posters, comfortable chairs and stuff. So it doesn't feel like a classroom. So it feels like a learning place.

I am. When I can is, I can be. When I be, I can learn. I am.

REFERENCES

Alonso, G., Anderson, N. S., Su, C., & Theoharis, J. (2009). *Our schools suck: Students talk back to a segregated nation on the failures of urban education.* New York, NY: NYU Press.

Anderson, K. S. (2009). *War or common cause? A critical ethnography of language education policy, race, and cultural citizenship.* Charlotte, NC: Information Age.

Ayers, W. C., Quinn, T., & Stovall, D. (2007). *Handbook for social justice in education.* New York, NY: Routledge.

Behar, R. (1996). *The vulnerable observer: Anthropology that breaks your heart.* Boston, MA: Beacon Press.

Brown, A. L., Crowley, R. M., & King, L. J. (2011). Black civitas: An examination of Carter Woodson's contributions to Teaching about race, citizenship, and the black soldier. *Theory and Research in Social Education, 39*(2), 278–299.

Brown, K. D., & Brown, A. L. (2010). Silenced memories: An examination of the sociocultural knowledge on race and racial violence in official school curriculum. *Equity & Excellence in Education, 43*(2), 139–154. doi:10.1080/10665681003719590

Caponi, G. D. (Ed.). (1999). *Signifyin(g), sanctifyin', & slam dunking: A reader in African American expressive culture.* Amherst, MA: University of Massachusetts Press.

Cooper, A. J. (1892). *A voice from the South, by a Black woman from the South.* Retrieved from, http://docsouth.unc.edu/church/cooper/cooper.html

Davis, B., & Sumara, D. (2006). *Complexity and education: Inquiries into learning, teaching, and research.* Mahwah, NJ: Lawrence Erlbaum.

Delpit, L. (2006). *Other people's children: Cultural conflict in the classroom.* New York, NY: New Press.

Dewey, J. (1998). *Art as experience.* New York, NY: Perigree. (Original work published 1934)

Dewey, J. (1929). *Experience and nature.* London, England: George Allen & Unwin.

Delpit, L. (1995). *Other people's children: Cultural conflict in the classroom.* New York, NY: New Press.

Delpit, L. (2013). *Multiplication is for white people": Raising expectations for other people's children.* New York, NY: New Press.

Donald, D. (2009, Spring). Forts, curriculum, and indigenous: Imagining decolonization of Aboriginal-Canadian relations in educational contexts. *First Nations Perspectives: The Journal of the Manitoba First Nations Education Resource Centre, 2*(1), 1–24. Retrieved from http://www.mfnerc.org/images

Dubois, W.E.B. (1903). *The souls of Black folk.* New York, NY: Bantam Classic.

DuBois, W.E.B. (1926). "Criteria of negro art." Retrieved from http://www.webdubois.org/db CriteriaNArt.html

Classen, C. (1993). *Worlds of sense: Exploring the senses across cultures.* New York, NY: Routledge.

Clough, P. T., & Halley, J. (2007). *The affective turn: Theorizing the social.* Durham, NC: Duke University Press.

Erlmann, V. (2010). *Reason and resonance: A history of modern aurality.* Cambridge, MA: Zone Books.

Gershon, W. S. (2011). Introduction: Towards a sensual curriculum. [Special Issue: Sensual Curriculum]. *Journal of Curriculum Theorizing, 27*(2), 1–16.

Gershon, W. S. (2012). Troubling notions of risk: Dissensus, dissonance, and making sense of students and learning. *Critical Studies in Education, 53*(3), 361–373.

Gershon, W. S. (2013). Vibrational affect: Sound theory and practice in qualitative research. *Cultural Studies ↔ Critical Methodologies, 13*(4), 257–262.

Gershon, W. S. (2017a). *Sound curriculum: Sonic studies in educational theory, method & practice.* New York, NY: Routledge.

Gershon W. S. (2017b). *Curriculum and students in classrooms: Everyday urban education in an era of standardization.* Lanham, MD: Lexington Books.

Geurts, K. L. (2002). *Culture and the senses: Bodily ways of knowing in an African community.* Berkeley, CA: University of California Press.

Gottlieb, A., & Graham, P. (1994). *Braided worlds.* Chicago, IL: University of Chicago Press.

Grande, S. (2004). *Red pedagogy: Native American social and political thought.* Lanham, MD: Rowman & Littlefield.

Gregg, M., & Seigworth, G. J. (Eds.). (2010). *The affect theory reader.* Durham, NC: Duke University Press.

Helfenbein, R. J. (2009). Thinking through scale: Critical geography and curriculum spaces. In E. Malewski (Ed.), *Curriculum studies handbook: The next moment* (pp. 304–317). New York, NY: Routledge.

Hemmings, C. (2006). Invoking affect. *Cultural studies, 19*(5), 548–567.

Howes, D. (2003). *Sensual relations: Engaging the senses in culture & social theory.* Ann Arbor, MI: University of Michigan Press.

Howes, D. (Ed.). (2009). *The sixth sense reader.* Oxford, England: Berg Press.

Janks, H. (2007). *Literacy and power.* New York, NY: Routledge.

Kliebard, H. M. (2004). *The struggle for the American curriculum, 1893–1958* (3rd ed.). New York, NY: Routledge.

Lipman, P. (1998). *Race, class, and power in school restructuring*. Albany, NY: State University of New York Press.

Lather, P. A., & Smithies, C. S. (1997). *Troubling the angels: Women living with HIV/AIDS*. Boulder, CO: Westview Press.

Massumi, B. (2002). *Parables for the virtual: Movement, affect, sensation*. Durham, NC: Duke University Press.

Massumi, B. (2011). *Semblance and event: Activist philosophy and the occurent arts*. Cambridge, MA: MIT Press.

McDermott, R., & Aron, J. (1978). Pirandello in the classroom: On the possibility of equal educational opportunity in American culture. In M. Reynolds (Ed.). *Futures of education*. Reston, VA: Council on Exceptional Children.

McNeil, L. (2000). *Contradictions of school reform: Educational costs of standardized testing*. New York, NY: Routledge.

Mehan, H. (1979). "What time is it Denise?": Asking known information questions in classroom discourse. *Theory into Practice, 18*, 285–294.

Mills, C. W. (1998). *Blackness visible: Essays on philosophy and race*. Ithaca, NY: Cornell University Press.

Ng-A-Fook, N. (2007). *An Indigenous curriculum of place: The United Houma Nation's contentious relationship with Louisiana's educational institutions*. New York, NY: Peter Lang.

Pennington, J. L. (2005). *The colonization of literacy education: A story of reading in one elementary school*. New York, NY: Peter Lang.

Readings, B. (1996). *The university in ruins*. Cambridge, MA: Harvard University Press.

Rist, R. C. (1973). *The urban school: A factory of failure*. Cambridge, MA: MIT Press.

Roelofs, M. (Ed.). (2009). Aesthetics and race: New philosophical perspectives. *Contemporary Aesthetics [Special Volume 2]*. Retrieved from https://contempaesthetics.org/newvolume/pages/journal.php?volume=41

Schubert, W. H. (1985). *Curriculum, perspective, and possibility*. Boston, MA: Allyn & Bacon.

Sedgwick, E. K. (2003). *Touching feeling: Affect, pedagogy, performance*. Durham, NC: Duke University Press.

Stewart, K. (2007). *Ordinary affects*. Durham, NC: Duke University Press.

Stoller, P. (1997). *Sensuous scholarship*. Philadelphia, PA: University of Pennsylvania Press.

Taubman, P. M. (2009). *Teaching by numbers: Deconstructing the discourse of standards and accountability in education*. New York, NY: Routledge.

Tsing, A. L. (2005). *Friction: An ethnography of global connection*. Princeton, NJ: Princeton University Press.

Tsing, A. L. (2015). *The mushroom at the end of the world: On the possibility of life in capitalist ruins*. Princeton, NJ: Princeton University Press.

Valencia, R. R. (Ed.). (1997). *The evolution of deficit thinking: Educational thought and practice*. London, England and Washington, DC: Falmer.

Valencia, R. R. (Ed.). (2010). *Dismantling contemporary deficit thinking: Educational thought and practice*. New York, NY: Routledge.

Valenzuela, A. (Ed.). (2005). Leaving children behind: How "Texas-style" accountability fails Latinoyouth. New York, NY: State University of New York Press.

Varenne, H., & McDermott, R. (1998). *Successful failure: The schools America builds*. Boulder, CO: Westview Press.

Valli, L., Croninger, R. G., Chambliss, M. H., Graeber, A. O., & Buese, D. (2008). *Test driven: High-stakes accountability in elementary schools*. New York, NY: Teachers College.

Watkins, W. H. (2001). *The White architects of Black education: Ideology and power in America, 1865–1954*. New York, NY: Teachers College Press.

Watkins, W. H. (Ed.). (2011). *The assault on public education: Confronting the politics of corporate school reform*. New York, NY: Teachers College Press.

Wills, J. (2006). Authority, culture, context: Controlling the production of historical knowledge in elementary classrooms. In J. L. Pace & A. Hemmings (Eds.), *Classroom authority: Theory, research, and practice* (pp. 33–62). Mahwah, NJ: Erlbaum.

Winfield, A. G. (2007). *Eugenics and education in America: Institutional racism and the implication of history, ideology, and memory*. New York, NY: Peter Lang.

Woodson, C. G. (1933). *The mis-education of the Negro*. Retrieved from http://www.historyisaweapon.com/defcon1/misedne.html

CHAPTER 9

(UN)BOXING THE SENSES

Curricular Practices of Sensory Ethnography

Kimberly Powell and Susan Uhlig
The Pennsylvania State University

9 March, 2015: Along the Wien Walking Path: Sue Uhlig

As I looked toward my chosen path in Central Park, from where I stood in Freedman Plaza that housed Tatiana Trouve's *Desire Lines* to the Wien Walk,[1] I felt somewhat lost in that I didn't know what to expect on my short walk, and I didn't know what to focus my senses on. As part of a field assignment for a course in sensory ethnography, I engaged in this walk to consider ways in which sensory experiences of place could be collected, experienced, performed, and materialized as affective responses of defamiliarization that would disrupt everyday assumptions, habits, and engagements.

What sense do I privilege? Sight? There were many things to look at: signs, people walking, people sitting, people talking, people working, vendor booths, trees, snow, puddles, objects on the ground. Sound? The cacophony of an urban area was complex: construction noises, vehicles moving along Fifth Avenue and 60th Street, car horns, people talking, people walking, birds chirping, carts rolling on the cobblestones, the music

Sensuous Curriculum:
Politics and the Senses in Education, pp. 157–174

coming from the clock. Smell? No particular smell stood out to me in the Park, which is strange since I am always affected by the smells walking along the city streets. I passed two food carts, but I didn't smell either one. I passed through the zoo, but didn't smell any animals. The only smell that stood out to me was fresh, of the cold humidity of melting snow.

Touch? While I didn't physically touch everything on my walk, I experienced tactile sensations of movement on the pavers, walking on snow and in puddles, and in picking up cold, damp, objects with my bare hands as I strolled on the Wien Walk. My walk was a purposefully slow saunter in which I purposely attended to my own perception as I moved through the space of Central Park. I looked all around; up to the blue sky, down on the melting snow on the pavers, at the bustling activity along the path, across the path to a nearby path, over at the looming buildings of the city, and back to where I began. I collected six objects as I walked the path. Collecting objects during the sensory walk was an important facet of the walk, because I wanted to experience a tactile understanding of public space. The melting snow that lined the path created soggy conditions for object collection, so I looked for objects that were made of non-porous materials, such as glass, plastic, and metal. The objects that glimmered in the sunlight in particular caught my attention.

During this walk, I questioned not only how I understand place but also what it means to be in place with others, imaginatively and relationally, in a shared space of informal learning: How do I capture and communicate my sensorial experience of place? I conceived of this walk as an imaginative conversation of meaning-making with place, objects, and others within an assemblage. My body collected sensory data as I moved through space within a structured time, and additional data was recorded via camera, audio recording, and found objects. In order to record the data, I "boxed" it up, with the box becoming a literal receptacle of my sensed experiences. While creative thought is said to exist outside the box, I find that having materials contained inside a box allows me to perform more nuanced problem solving of carefully curated thought, precisely because the very borders of the box delineated moments of experience and engagement, drawing attention to the object by literally framing it within a new context. The box acts as a framework to provide a structure which organizes my research, ideas, and experiences in an aesthetic composition while still allowing for fluidity of arrangement.

A PEDAGOGY OF SENSORIAL ENCOUNTER: KIMBERLY POWELL

Sue's above-described encounter with her walk and subsequent exhibit emerged from a graduate course that I designed and taught in the spring of

2015 entitled "Sensory Ethnography." As the course instructor, I sought to experiment with form and format alongside my students, so that the course had an emergent, experimental and open-ended quality to it rather than a predesigned set of course objectives. While sensory ethnography is largely anchored in the social sciences and their corresponding methodological approaches (e.g., interviews, participant observation), at the heart of our pursuit were the ways in which art practices might prominently function in, for, and as sensory research. Art and research share similar practices: both require, for example, the development of attentiveness to and attunement with rendering the familiar strange and the strange familiar (e.g., Spindler & Spindler, 1982). Increasingly, qualitative researchers have acknowledged and argued for epistemological and ontological stances toward research as an emergent, relational event in which research design, inquiry, and analysis remain responsive to sensorial, material, affective (e.g., precognitive, "felt" forces) encounters (St. Pierre, 2014; Truman & Springgay, 2016; Throughout the course, this relationship between art and research was underscored and blurred. So, too, were the distinctions between art and everyday practices. In many ways, the fieldwork experiences prompted all of us in the course to think about how everyday life—its practices, activities, and social arrangements—might be considered artful and experimental in the Deweyan sense of experience as something comprised of both doing and undergoing (Dewey, 1938). Sue Uhlig's experience and experimentation with sensory ethnography, as described above and throughout this chapter, perform sensory encounters of ethnographic fieldworking.

Over the course of the semester, we explored several theories, methods, and ethnographies that situated, inspired and framed individual student fieldworking in ways that were open-ended and experimental. Readings came from a variety of fields and standpoints but clustered around three considerations. First, we read anthropological essays and cross-cultural fieldwork of the senses and perception, stressing the senses as culturally constructed categories that are imbued with social values (e.g., Howes, 2005; Stoller, 1989). Many of the readings emphasized intersensoriality, synaesthesia, and a critical interrogation into assumptions about what the senses are and do, thus destabilizing our assumptions about the social order of things as encountered through perception. Theories of intersensoriality and synesthesia, for example, are suggestive of the connections and resonances inherent in multiple sources of sensations that link bodily experiences to thought and action as perceiver and perceived blur (e.g., Connor, 2008; Feld, 2005; Powell, 2010). As a case study, we read Oliver Sacks' cases of visual experiences in blinded people and his argument for the interconnectedness and interactions of the sensory areas in the brain, of in-between states, the "intersensory" or "metamodel" (2005, p. 33).

A second significant aspect of the course pedagogy is the concept of sensory ethnography as an embodied practice of being *with*—in participation, or in shared or imaginative empathy with others—which calls for engagement with the practices of everyday life (Pink, 2011). We read and worked with ethnographic methods of attunement and emplacement (the interrelationship of body, mind, and environment), such as everyday practices of walking, talking, and eating as a means of engaging and evoking the sensory and affective dimensions of experiences (De Certeau, 1984; Pink, 2009). For some students in the class, like Sue, Pink's (2009) contention that "the self emerges from the process of sensory learning, being shaped through a person's engagement with the social, sensory and material environment of which she or he is a part" (p. 40) was an essential part of framing their fieldworking experiences. We also discussed some of the roots of this work as seen, for example, in Paul Stoller's (1997) idea of ethnographic fieldwork as sensuous methodology, a means to encourage participation in a variety of cultural practices and render more vividly the worlds of others.

A third dimension of sensory scholarship and pedagogy that is addressed in the course includes theories from posthumanism and new materialism, which hold views of sensation as something unfolding and vague rather than constituted by a particular form (Massumi, 2011) and emphasize the agency and materiality of human and non-human actants (Bennett, 2010). All of these concepts emphasize practices of intersensorial and material relations that are always unfolding in process—an event, precognitive in the sense that it registers first as affect, as a felt force on and in the body before it is registered at a conscious level. Pertaining to the senses, for example, Massumi (2011) argues for amodality rather than cross-modality as a means of understanding what happens between the senses rather than what is registering within a particular sense (e.g., seeing or hearing). While cross-modality refers to multiple senses being involved in an experience wherein one sense might also evoke another, amodality refers to perception of a particular event as not actually being in any particular mode of sensory perception, thus remaining "virtual," as a "lived abstraction" (p. 18): we might recompose our senses for any particular event so that something we think of as dominantly visual might actually be recomposed as dominantly aural, or tactile. Similarities across sensory experiences bring forth what he refers to as a "self-organizing of experience" (p. 111), where a certain affective quality resonates. Massumi refers to this particular quality as a vitality affect, which gives rise to forms of life that are shared.

When Sue describes (above) her Wein walk and subsequent curatorial experience in terms of how the boxes provide her with both a framework to organize and delineate her "research, ideas, and experiences" and allow her "to perform more nuanced problem-solving for carefully curated thought" we might be led at first be led to think these boxes are separating and dividing sensory encounters. Her acknowledgement, however, that the boxes "delineated moments of experience" into "aesthetic compositions" that allow for fluidity of recomposition underscores Massumi's (2011) notion of the virtual inherent in any experience, as it suggests that her perception of her sensory experience with walking might be continually recomposed and rearranged. Her walking and artist boxes underscore and illuminate the processes that we undergo with amodality and the virtual in everyday experience. Further, the concept of the virtual suggests felt extensions (p. 106) of the visual, tactile, and so forth: perceptual feeling without *actual*, literal perception that is nonetheless experienced as perception of the event. This is also how sensory fieldwork as a curricular encounter is living and emergent.

SENSORY FIELDWORKING AND TECHNIQUES

In order to enact the course philosophy and approach of sensory ethnography, the fieldwork assignments were intentionally left open to experimentation, play, and choice. Powell dedicated much of the course to fieldworking experiences in the senses that were inspired by the readings and by several artists working in the domain of the senses. These explorations intentionally disrupted the taken-for-granted in everyday practices such as eating, walking, or listening/sounding in order to produce and encounter new relations of sensory experiences. The fieldwork exercises pertained to vision/image, hearing/sound/vibration, touch/materialization, kinesthesia/ambulation/vibration, taste/food, and smell/scent. At first glance, these exercises divide the senses and appear to reify a Western categorization of the senses and sensory engagement. In practice, however, each sensory exercise served to underscore and perform the amodal nature of sensory engagement.

Powell structured each of the exercises in a similar manner with several choices made available to students. For each exercise, students were encouraged to create their own fieldwork exercise, either through "riffing" off of the assignment structure or by creating something wholly new. The open-ended nature of the assignments were, in fact, meant to emphasize the ways in which artists experimentally engage with material, sensory, and embodied encounters as part of art practice. In many cases, as is the case with Sue's artful play, students would extend, create, and/or depart entirely from the choices they had with each assignment. The interplay between structure/order/system and differentiation/disruption/riffing that Powell put into play was largely informed through her background in music pedagogy, specifically that of jazz training which alternates between structure and improvisation. Pedagogically and ontologically, Powell was also informed through the work of Deleuze and his major concepts that perform the idea of life which requires a form of order and system and "that which also opens the system" (Colebrook, 2010, p. 5)

The pedagogy and curriculum for the course became emergent and relational. Each week, following these fieldwork assignments, students would then share in class their ethnographic pursuits. This activity allowed for multiple opportunities. First, the sharing of this work created the space for reflection on what students had done, which was useful for revisions or new ideas based on feedback. Second, students grasped the inherent multiplicity of any given choice—even when students chose the exact same assignment option, the possible processes, experiences and outcomes were varied and unpredictable.

Third, beyond reflection, this sharing became an event (Deleuze, 1993), defined as changes that are immanent (both real or possible) within a particular confluence of forces; it is the potential for transformation that is incorporeal and moves above any particular space and time; it is dynamism inherent in the actualization of any activity (Stagoll, 2010, p. 89). The sharing of fieldwork in class was an occasion for the performativity of sensory data: as students shared their fieldwork, the material became *dynamic* an occasion for new insight, impromptu experimentation, improvisation, and possibility. Importantly, Deleuze's concept of the event constitutes disruption. The assigned sensory fieldwork that is then shared in class functions as a disruption, a "dislocation of thinking" (Colebrook 2010, p. 4) regarding, in our case, expectations marking pedagogy, curriculum, and qualitative research.

What follows in the remainder of this chapter is a condensed description of the sensory fieldwork exercises Powell gave to students during the course and Uhlig's experimentation with fieldwork as sensory experience. As such, this is a comparatively rare chance to consider classroom interactions from the perspective of both teacher and student, an opportunity that also makes explicit the multisensuous interrelations of an event from multiple perspectives.

Vision/Image

Please choose between five possible explorations: (1) observe an activity, a place, or an object and engage in *connected detachment* (a methodological practice of working simultaneously subjectivity and objectivity, developed in Bresler, 2013) to imagine seeing it for the first time; (2) engage in a familiar activity or visit a familiar place, but take someone unfamiliar with it and write their perspective; (3) blindfold yourself and move about in a familiar place to encourage thinking about vision in a different way; (4) use a visual method, such as mapping or photo-elicitation, and specific prompt with a participant; (5) invent your own method of inquiry, and/or use some combination of the above

Hearing/Sound/Vibration

For the sound exploration fieldwork, consider the readings and discussion pertaining to acoustemology, soundscapes and aural ecology (e.g., Atkinson, 2006; Feld, 2005; Rice, 2005). You could choose between five possible explorations: (1) observe the aural ecology of a space/place/activity to examine, for example, potential "acoustics of power" (Rice, 2005, p. 8) constructed through sound; (2) listening while not seeing, making sense of the ways in which sound spatially arranges place; (3) creating a sound collage, journal or walk via found sounds; or, (4) create a life narrative comprising music and text; (5) invent your own method of inquiry, and/or use some combination of the above.

Taste/Food and Smell/Scent

Choose between the taste and smell assignments or combined in some way. You could create a scent map or scentscape describing the places and scents associated with them, create a scent. You could choose from the following: (1) The Art of Scent teaching packet prepared by the Museum of Art and Design, choose an activity that is suggested in the readings (Pankow, 2012, pp. 11–13: Activity 1.1–1.4) and adapt these exercises as you see fit to your own context; 2). create, or have a participant create, a scent map of "scentscape"; create a scent biography in which someone describes their life experiences through smells and the various associations, social and cultural practices, and memories that certain smells call forth.

For the taste exercise, you could engage in the following: (1) Engage in a walking tour and interview with a friend, roommate, partner, child; (2) prepare or have someone prepare a meal for you and engage in conversation that pertains to the meal (e.g., associated memories, cooking techniques); (3) Engage in a "tasting" either at home or at an eating establishment(s) with a friend, roommate, partner, child; (4) Engage in a mindful eating exercise. Eat in silence and engage in eating as if you are doing it for the very first time. Or, invent your own method of inquiry, or use some combination of the above.

Kinesthesia/Ambulation/Vibration

For the kinaesthetic/ambulatory inquiry, students explored walking and movement as inquiry. Options included taking a walk with a neighbor, friend, or child and asking them to give a tour of their neighborhood; incorporating elements of play and chance in a walk, after artists that engage in those techniques; walking with a young child and following their lead, path, and activity; engaging in a soundwalk; and walking with someone who navigates with an assistive device (e.g., wheelchair, skateboard, crutches, stroller) to understanding pathways, obstacles, opportunities, and experiences; and, creating their own walk or movement-oriented inquiry.

Touch/Materialization/Tactility/Texture

Based on the article concerning clay impressions (http://hyperallergic.com/195077/impressions-of-new-york-city-streets-captured-in-clay/), which encourages us to think about clay as a "conduit between people and place", we will first make clay together as a class as a material encounter. Then, on your own, you will take make a clay impression of an aspect of a place (e.g., materials in that place) that holds meaning for you in some way: a place that fascinates you, scares you, and/or holds your attention in some way, attending to the textures and what the textures cause you to (re)experience about that place.

SENSORY BOXES OF PEDAGOGICAL SPACES: SUE'S FIELDWORK

With the knowledge that there would be a total of five sensory assignments, I decided to unify all assignments with a structured box format, beginning with the first one on Vision/Image. For each exercise, I focused on my sensorial experience of interacting with others in spaces I consider public and pedagogical, spaces in which a public collective can gather, interact, and/or move that shape understandings of culture, such as museums, streets, and city squares (e.g., Hickey, 2010). To guide me as I worked on the series, I used Pink's (2009) description of sensory ethnography, which she describes as an "emergent" (p. 9) and "critical methodology" (p. 8) that "involves the researcher self-consciously and reflexively attending to the senses throughout the research process, that is during the planning, reviewing, fieldwork, analysis, and representational processes of a project" in order to represent and generate new knowledge based on experience (p. 10). Accordingly, as I further detail in this section, I adapted and refined my methodology throughout the processes of fieldworking and box creation.

In the making of these sensory boxes, I questioned how I came to understand place through the senses by documenting my encounters, with an aim to provoke discussion with others in the sensory ethnography class and potentially beyond.

Documentation of each site consisted of notes I jotted down in a notebook and photographs I took, most frequently with my iPhone and only occasionally with a DSLR camera due to its bulky size. As I collected this visual and written data, I increasingly found value in also collecting material objects to place inside each box as tactile data, These objects provided a physical, material dimension to expand how sensory experiences are communicated and shared—they are one way to render the discursively theoretical, concrete.

To create the series of boxes, I used a set of 7" x 5" x 1.75" lidded cardboard boxes from a beauty subscription company. Inside each partitioned box were layers of content that emphasize the material and emplaced nature of my sensory experiences. When the box lid is first opened, the first layer encountered contains 32 photocards that each measure 4.25" x 5.5," a similar size and format of postcards which allude to implied correspondence and the ephemerality of place. One side of the photocards depicted a photographic image as a visual documentation of place while the other side contained the correspondence, or the textual narration of sensual experiences that address place and time. Underneath the stack of photocards were maps I drew on acetate sheets of the places in which the events of the box occurred. Only a few pieces of cartographical information, such as paths walked and places visited, was marked on the clear acetate sheets, so that the contents on the bottom of the boxes can be seen peeking through the transparent parts of each visual map. Last, nestled within dividers at the base of the box are two to nine found objects collected at each site. The types of objects I chose to collect were emergent and depended on the fieldworking site; I chose shiny, non-porous materials in the melting snow of Central Park and food related items in New Orleans.

The collections at the bottom of the boxes evoke artist assemblage boxes, such as those by mid 20th century artist Joseph Cornell. They also resemble the format of a *wunderkammer* (German "wonder room") and imply a cabinet of curiosities or collector's cabinet (Hooper-Greenhill, 1992). *Wunderkammer* could be a box, a cabinet, or an entire room that is dedicated to housing a variety of objects in categories such as natural history, ethnography, geology, religion, and art. According to art historian Arthur Wheelock (1998), the 16th-century scholar Samuel Quiccheberg supported the idea of collections, and in his ideal museum, artwork such as prints and drawings would be collected in addition to natural history and ethnographic items because these objects "provided knowledge important in man's quest for a virtuous life" (p. 35). Dutch artist Rembrandt van Rijn found it critical to collect *artificialia*, objects made by human hand, and *naturalia*, organic objects, to inform his intellect and to include as props and inspiration within his paintings (Tissink, 2003). In my sensory boxes, I include both *naturalia* and *artificialia* in found objects and art in a quest not for providing knowledge but to facilitate knowledge in the making as multisensory approach to placemaking.

What follows are descriptions of each of the five boxes. The order they are appear in this chapter are the order in which they were created.

Sensory Boxes of Pedagogical Spaces: Vision

The *Sensory Box of Pedagogical Spaces: Vision* centers on the visuality and performativity of a ceramic demonstration and workshop held on my university campus during a daylong event. The morning event was set in the ceramics studio, where Nigerian ceramic artist Ibukunoluwa Ayoola , also known as IBK, conducted an artist demonstration on the potter's wheel. The partnering afternoon event was located nearby in Reservoir Studio, a small studio in one of the oldest buildings on campus. Art Education professor B. Stephen Carpenter founded Reservoir Studio as a way for a collective to take pedagogical action, whose main project is the "collaborative creative resistance of the global water crisis and the enactment of research, design, production, and public education of point of use ceramic water filters as art/curriculum to promote adequate access to potable water" (Reservoir Studio, About). During the water filter workshop, potter Richard Wukich and IBK joined Carpenter to demonstrate how to make point of use filters, and all others in attendance were encouraged to participate in making clay for the filters. My primary interest in fieldworking during the demonstration/workshop was to explore the shifts between being a passive observer during an artist demonstration while being an active participant-observer in the water filter workshop. At both partnering events, I took written notes and dozens of photos, both on my iPhone and DSLR camera. From the workshop, I collected sawdust and powdered clay, which provide additional sensory experiences in smell and touch. As participant in the workshop, I was immersed in the participatory and multisensory experience of making, which shifted my ability to observe, take photos, and jot down notes. Below is text from one of the thirty-two photocards, which is set in the studio workshop.

Card 14. 23 January 2015 3:13 p.m. Reservoir Studio

The larger screens are also used to create the sawdust. Upon Steve's return at 3:30, the production of sawdust making speeds up. Two different stations of sawdust making are called to action. I am at one station with Steve and another student. We use this larger screen to make as much sawdust as we can. The wood shavings smell like hamster bedding. The wood is jagged and uneven. Pressing the wood against the screen hurts my hand as individual wood pieces jab my hand. The smell of the wood and the shavings reminds me of my dad, who was a cabinetmaker. A flood of emotions comes over me, but I restrain them and redirect my focus back to the mission of the water filters.

Sensory Boxes of Pedagogical Spaces: Sound

The *Sensory Box of Pedagogical Spaces: Sound* centered on the auditory experiences of my visit to the Miniature Railroad & Village at the Carnegie Science Center in Pittsburgh, Pennsylvania on 2/13/15 after I finished my duties as student teaching supervisor in the Pittsburgh Public Schools. While model trains have never interested me, I took advantage of a friend's offer to provide a tour of the Railroad and Village, and it seemed a good time to explore the aural ecology of the exhibit. The space, filled with moving model trains and mechanized animations, was noisy on its own. Added to those base sounds were the chatter of visitors, the songs of children, the occasional train whistle, and digital noises from adjacent museum spaces, which provided a layered cacophony in which to tune in and tune out. During the tour and while on my own in the exhibition, I detailed observances, jotted visitor conversations, and charted times on an exhibition map of the display. I recorded the tour and general sounds in the exhibition using the Voice Record app on my iPhone. I also took photos of the model train village and the storage area, in the general exhibit and on particular features that my guide pointed out to me. I spent time listening to the trains and visitors. The adults I observed identified the building or event names authoritatively and also reminisced about the buildings while the children made up songs or expressed verbal delight with the trains and animations. Because I spent 2.5 hours in the museum exhibit, I had hours of recorded sound to transcribe, hundreds of photos to examine, and pages of written notes. My friend and tour guide also gave me a dozen artifacts from the model village storage area. It was the most difficult box to curate since I had so much data to work with. I matched the photos up with transcriptions and my descriptions of the site. What I ultimately selected was based on aesthetic and narrative choices, of what pairings of images and text made for the most compelling storytelling. Object selection was similar in determining the best visual assemblage.

Admittedly, the acoustemology in this site was difficult to capture in the box format. Textually, I described the soundscapes of each site on the photocards, which included conversations and place specific sounds. However, as Feld (2005) notes, there is a temporality of the acousemology of place. He writes, "as a sensual space-time, the experience of place potentially can always be grounded in an acoustic dimension" (p. 185). Since portraying pedagogical places through the sensorium was integral to my research, I was determined to ground my experience of place through the fleeting quality of sound, at least in two of the boxes where the soundscapes were of particular importance. In addition to the photocards, map, and collected objects, I also include a small battery operated recording device on which I recorded the sound of the train whistle heard in the Miniature Railroad and Village. Sound could also be activated by shaking the box through the looseness of the objects on the bottom layer of each box. Outside of the physical confines of the box, I also uploaded place-based sounds to Soundcloud.

Card 18. February 2015 1:30–3:30 p.m. Miniature Railroad & Village

Hear 1 minute 25 seconds of sounds from this section on Soundcloud: Railroad and Village soundscape 18.[2] *This is a general recording of exhibition and visitor sounds. I am close to the train whistle, so its sound is clear. The corner of the exhibit has drawn a crowd. Layered voices talk about Forbes field, with distinct conversations partially obscured by the train whistle and a passing train. A young child sings, "Choo-choo!" A man is eager to talk about Forbes field, and identifies such things as the shape of the grass. A boy exclaims, "Mom, look at second base." He repeats it until his mom responds. On my tour, Sarah tells me that there are 23,000 spectators in the stadium made of hand painted Q-tips.*

Sensory Boxes of Pedagogical Spaces: Smell and Taste

For the *Sensory Boxes of Pedagogical Spaces: Smell and Taste*, I documented my experiences with taste and smell at seven different restaurants and food shops in New Orleans, Louisiana over four days while I attended a conference located in the city. New Orleans is a city associated with good food, good music, and a good time. In this box, I set out to explore the sense of taste in New Orleans in the Warehouse District, the Central Business District, and the French Quarter. In reading Lisa Heldke's (2005) chapter, "But is it Authentic?," I contemplated the idea of eating as "a kind of conversation" (p. 389) in which the food, the preparer, and the eater engage in a dialogue, each bringing their unique contributions, perspectives, and experiences. The conversation shifts when the patron is a cultural outsider. Heldke writes, "the work of cuisine is a different work for the cultural insider than it is for the cultural tourist" (p. 389). For cultural outsiders, what is the authentic New Orleans experience? What should it be?

To continue the involvement of incorporating relational dialogue into my project, I used the suggestions of others, a mixture of cultural insiders and outsiders, to determine where and what I should eat in New Orleans.

First, I crowd sourced suggestions for restaurants on social media, which led to my eating dinner at an acclaimed Cajun restaurant. Then, I searched on Trip Advisor for the "best food in New Orleans," and a candy shop topped the list. When I got to New Orleans on the first day, I asked the airport shuttle bus driver for his suggestions, and his recommendation led to a group of us going to seafood restaurant in the French Quarter that specialized in fried foods. During a preconference workshop, the artist who conducted the workshop offered suggestions on where to eat lunch, which led to my experience at a nearby deli. Once at the restaurants and candy shop, I asked the servers for their recommendations, often taking their exact suggestions. During my experiences at each place, I took photographs with my iPhone, wrote in my notebook, and collected objects, such as candy, fortune cookie fortune, plastic piece, paper napkin holder, plastic stir stick, broken Mardi Gras bead necklace, and paper Easter grass. I told only one server, the cashier at the candy shop, of my purpose in collecting objects. Upon hearing my project, she excitedly gathered a few items for me, let me take her photo, and freely chatted with me about her experiences in working at the candy shop. Since this box focused on taste and smell, I felt implored to add food. It is the only box with edible content.

Card 21. 3 March 2015, 10:10–10:40 a.m. Candy shop

Have I mentioned the sweet smell wafting through the entire space? The candy shop is a relatively small space. There are two entrances to the shop, and both entrances have a candy making area where candy is constantly being made in full view of patrons. The south entrance is where the pralines and candied nuts are made, and all other candies are made in by the north entrance. In between the candy production areas is the shop where patrons can choose from packaged goods, some candies made on site, and some are imported locally and regionally. There's an area for ice cream. And there's the candy counter, where there are dozens of candies to choose from. All of this sugar that fills the environment is sweet but not sickly sweet. I was in the space for 30 minutes, and I did not get tired of the smell nor did it linger on my clothes or in my hair. The space was brightly lit and pleasant. For being in a candy shop for 30 minutes, I generally felt welcome by the workers and by the space itself. One female candymaker helped me the most. She has worked at the candyshop for 7 years. I asked her if she ever tires of the sweet aroma, and she said she doesn't. She said the candy smell does linger on her clothes and body. "Dogs love me," she said.

Sensory Boxes of Pedagogical Spaces: Movement

In *Sensory Boxes of Pedagogical Spaces: Movement*, I focused on movement, place, and objects in response to a 3-day exploration of New York City that included a concert, museum visits, and time spent with family in Brooklyn. For this box, I centered on the interaction with the public artwork *Desire Lines* by artist Tatiana Trouve that I viewed on March 9, 2015. *Desire Lines* was a public art work located at 60th Street and Fifth Avenue in Central Park's Doris C. Freedman Plaza, and it consisted of 212 spools of cord of various thicknesses and colors installed on three large metal brackets. The lengths of cord on each spool corresponded to the distance on each of the 212 walking paths in Central Park. To more narrowly define the parameters of my box on movement, I carefully selected one spool from among the 212 in *Desire Lines*, labeled "P095 From Scholars' Gate to the Wien Walk leading to the Arsenal, *Les pas perdus*." Using a map in a Central Park application on my iPhone, I identified the location along where the 1/3-mile Wien Walk path began at Scholar's Gate, passed through the Central Park Zoo, and ended at the Arsenal. As I ambled for an hour along the 1/3-mile path, I thought about the experiences I had in New York City over those three days, such as a concert and multiple museum visits, which informed the present to make new associations and meanings. I documented my sensory walk through photography, written notes, audio recordings[3], and found objects that I collected on the path, such as an eyeglass lens, gold twist tie, and pressed penny. I also included a small map of Central Park I printed from Google Maps, on which I embroidered green thread to mark my movement along the walking path. In addition to the photocard text below, another part of this journey is described in the introduction of this chapter.

Card 13. 9 March 2015 Central Park Sensory Wien Walk

Sounds of the Walk: New York Central Park [Sensory] Wien Walk Soundscape 4

Reflection and inspiration: The Bjork exhibit at MoMA, March 9. During the narrative audio tour at the Bjork exhibition at MoMA, the narrator spoke of Bjork as mother-girl needing to "rearrange things into new and just forms ... patterns that would make the strong accept the weak as equals." As I walked on the regularity of the hexagonal cobblestones in the Wien Walk, I thought of this notion of pattern as equals.

Reflection and inspiration II: Vibrant Matter and Thing Power. In Vibrant Matter (2010), Jane Bennett describes a collection of things found on a street gutter grate after a storm as having "Thing Power"—"the curious ability of inanimate things to animate, to act, to produce effects dramatic and subtle" (p. 6). She saw this assemblage of objects—a dead rat, a glove, oak pollen, a stick of wood, and a bottle cap—as things, as being vibratory, of having presence and life. As I drove and walked through Brooklyn and Manhattan seeing the debris unearthed in the melting and retreating snow banks, I thought of their life force, their thing power and welcomed their vibrancy back from the long winter into the renewal of spring. Along my Central Park

Sensory Wien Walk, the materials I found shimmied with vibrancy and I collected their thing power for my sensory box.

OBJECT: Metal twist tie, found 12:24 p.m.

Sensory Boxes of Pedagogical Spaces: Touch

Sensory Boxes of Pedagogical Spaces: Touch is the last box I created. It centers on the tactile qualities within eight different architectural places of learning with which I interacted during April 9 to April 17, 2015. I considered the ways in which these pedagogical places contributed towards ontological understanding through contemplation of tactile interactions within the buildings. I incorporated different ways of feeling and touching by weaving written and tactile perspectives of how the buildings can be understood. Textual descriptions included historical context of the building, my observations in the school setting as participant-observer, and public school data for the K–12 schools obtained from the school district's website. I also asked eight people with whom I interacted in those eight buildings to write a short description on how the building they work in feels to them. Gathering a variety of histories, experiences, and perspectives of a place allowed me to understand and appreciate it more deeply than if I were to only consider my own interactions, particularly if those interactions were brief. Textural imagery included photographs of the outside and inside of each building. Textural descriptions also included two tactile impressions on an area of the building's exterior entryway, made in tooling foil by rubbing the foil with a paper stump and with a small ball of clay pushed onto the same part of the entryway. I documented how the eight buildings felt through photography, written notes, and impressions in tooling foil and dried, unfired clay.

Card 12. Tactile Places of Learning: Urban Elementary School, Inside

Rip. Glue. Layer. Scratch. Repeat. A lesson on decollage got my attention as 6th grade students were involved in the process of reverse collaging. Students were introduced to the art of Italian artist Mimmo Rotella who used the technique of decollage in his work, ripping posters off the walls in Rome and gluing them to canvas back in his studio. Students also watched a video of the process and were shown images of accidental decollages in Pittsburgh. Using magazines, glue sticks, scissors, and sandpaper, students worked on creating surprising new images by layers numerous sheets of selected magazine pages. The student teacher directed them to use at least four images in their final work that contained juxtaposition and a particular message. Students were encouraged to carefully rip the layers apart to reveal images below. Experimentation was also encouraged in slicing the images with scissors or sanding them down with

> *sandpaper. Some students had clear ideas of how they wanted their artwork to look. Some students were happy with experimenting and playing with the materials. Others needed prodding to start the process. I talked with one student, who was hesitant to start on his work, citing the lack of magazine choices was limiting his project. I suggested he see it as a challenge. A short time later, he paged through a magazine, shut it, and said there are no good images in there. I showed him how a few ok images put together had a great theme, and he went to work. Cut. Sand. Slice. Shred. Repeat.*

ENTANGLEMENT

Our passages, above, describe the ways in which sensory fieldwork constitutes a sensuous curriculum and pedagogy in the making. While each box in the series draws attention to one particular sense as its theme, other senses are evoked in the written, visual, and material field notes given that sensual emplacement does not occur in isolation. Here, we acknowledge the work of Stephen Feld (2005), who argued that "experiencing and knowing place ... can proceed through a complex interplay of the auditory and the visual, as well as through other intersensory perceptual processes" (p. 185) and of Sarah Pink (2009), whose work in domestic environments has also prompted her to write about environment as "constituted, experienced, understood, evaluated and maintained through all the senses" (p. 13); rather than dominated by one sensory modality. But we also consider the ways in which, more than just containers for collecting sensory data, Sue's experimentation with artistic boxes are aesthetic compositions that she—or we, as viewers—might literally or conceptually recompose and rearrange as her perception of her sensory experience with walking in places might also continually be recomposed and rearranged, beyond the actual event of walking and "boxing." This is the amodality and the virtual of which Massumi (2011) writes about concerning art as an event: perception as occurring between the senses rather than in any one particular sense, giving rise to a qualitative affect both of and beyond a particular art work that might also constitute a dislocation of thinking, a disruption of our daily habits of sensing and sense making. The pedagogical, public spaces upon which Sue concentrates in her series of sensory boxes are understood through an entanglement of the sensorium rather than dominated by one sensory modality. Photos, maps, audio recordings, and objects all contributed to coming to understand place through the performativity of multimodal sensory data. Walter Gershon (2001, p. 1) has written about the ways in which sensorial and sensuality are entangled in sociocultural contexts:

> From this perspective, how someone makes sense of her world is a fluid intersection of sociocultural norms and values, agency, identity, physiology,

awareness, and personal taste. In these ways, sensual understandings are located firmly in the paradox of human experience, intensely personal and unique yet inexorably informed by interlocking layers of local and less local sociocultural norms and values.

Go for a walk. Look, listen, hear, touch, taste, smell, write. Move fast or slow, sketch or write, record or compose. Take clay impressions. Note affect. Defamiliarize yourself with your surroundings. Experiment. Unbox.

NOTES

1. The Wien Walk is one of 212 public walking paths in New York City's Central Park.
2. To listen to audio from the sensory walk in SoundCloud, follow the link https://soundcloud.com/sue-uhlig/sets/railroad-and-village
3. To listen to audio from the sensory walk in Central Park on SoundCloud, follow the link https://soundcloud.com/sue-uhlig/sets/new-york-central-park-sensory

REFERENCES

Atkinson, P. (2006). *The aural ecology of the city: Sound, noise, and exclusion in the city*. University of Tasmania: HACRU Occasional Paper 5.

Bennett, J. (2010). *Vibrant matter: A political ecology of things*. Durham, NC: Duke University Press.

Bresler, L. (2013). Experiential pedagogies in research education: Drawing on engagement With artworks. In C. Stout (Ed.), *Teaching and learning emergent research methodologies in art education* (pp. 43–64). Reston, VA: National Art Education Association.

Colebrook, C. (2010). Introduction. In A. Parr (Ed.), *The Deleuze dictionary: Revised edition* (pp. 1–6). Edinburgh, Scotland: Edinburgh University Press.

Connor, S. (2008). The shakes: Conditions of tremor. *Senses & Society, 3*(2), 205–220.

Deleuze, G. (1993). *The fold: Leibniz and the baroque* (T. Conley, Trans.). Minneapolis: University of Minnesota Press.Dewey, J. (1938). *Experience and education*. New York, NY: Macmillan.

De Certeau, M. (1984). *The practice of everyday life*. Berkeley and Los Angeles, CA: University of California Press.

Feld, S. (2005). Places sensed, senses placed: Toward a sensuous epistemology of environments. In D. Howes (Ed.), *Empire of the senses: The sensual culture reader* (pp. 179–191). New York, NY: Berg.

Gershon, W. S. (2011). Introduction: Toward a sensual curriculum. *Journal of Curriculum Theorizing, 27*(2), 1–16.

Hickey, A. (2010). When the street becomes a pedagogue. In J. A. Sandlin, B. D. Schultz, & J. Burdick (Eds.), *Handbook of public pedagogy: Education and learning beyond schooling* (pp. 161–170). London, England: Routledge.

Heldke, L. (2005). But is it authentic?: Culinary travel and the search for the "genuine article". In C. Korsmeyer (Ed.) *The taste culture reader: Experiencing food and drink* (pp. 385–394). New York, NY: Berg.

Hooper-Greenhill, E. (1992). *Museums and the shaping of knowledge*. London, England: Routledge.

Howes, D. (2005). Introduction: Empires of the senses. In D. Howes (Ed.), *Empire of the senses: The sensual culture reader* (pp. 1–20). New York, NY: Berg.

Massumi, B. (2011). *Semblance and event: Activist philosophy and the occurrent arts*. Cambridge, MA: MIT Press.

Pankow, P. (2012). The art of scent 1889-2012: Teacher resource packet. Retrieved from https://madmuseum.org/sites/default/files/static/ed/The%20Art%20of%20Scent%20TRP_0.pdf

Pink, S. (2009). *Doing sensory ethnography*. Thousand Oaks, CA: SAGE.

Pink, S. (2011). Images, senses and applications: Engaging visual anthropology. *Visual Anthropology, 24*, 437–454.

Powell, K. (2010). Making sense of place: Mapping as a multisensory research method. *Qualitative Inquiry, 16*(7), 539–555.

Rice, T. (2003). *Soundselves: An acoustemology of sound and self in the Edinburgh Royal Infirmary. Anthropology Today 19*(4), 1–9.

Reservoir Studio. (n.d.) About. Retrieved from https://sites.psu.edu/reservoirstudio/insidethereservoir/about/

Sacks, O. (2005). The mind's eye: What the blind see. In D. Howes (Ed.), *Empire of the senses: The sensual culture reader* (pp. 25–42). New York, NY: Berg.

Spindler, G. D., & Spindler, L. (1982). Roger Harker and Schönhausen: From the familiar to the strange and back again. In G. D. Spindler (Ed.), *Doing the ethnography of schooling* (pp. 20–46). New York, NY: Holt, Rinehart & Winston.

St. Pierre, E. A. (2014). A brief and personal history of post qualitative research: Toward "Post Inquiry." *Journal of Curriculum Theorizing 30*(2), 2–19.

Stagoll, C. (2010). Event. In A. Parr (Ed.), *The Deleuze dictionary: Revised edition* (pp. 89–91). Edinburgh, Scotland: Edinburgh University Press.

Stoller, P. (1989). *The taste of ethnographic things: The senses in anthropology*. Philadelphia, PA: University of Pennsylvania Press.

Stoller, P. (1997). *Sensuous scholarship*. Philadelphia, PA: University of Pennsylvania Press.

Tissink, F. (2003). *The Rembrandt house museum Amsterdam*. Ghent: Ludion.

Truman, S., & Springgay, S. (2016). Propositions for walking research. In P. Burnard, E. Mackinlay & K. Powell (Eds.), *The Routledge international handbook of intercultural arts research* (pp. 259–267). London, England: Routledge.

Wheelock, A. (1998). *A collector's cabinet*. Washington, DC: National Gallery of Art.

CHAPTER 10

SENSUOUS AND ARTISTIC CURRICULUM TOWARDS THE DISRUPTION OF THE NORMATIVE

Anniina Suominen
Aalto University

I truly believe that artistic knowledge and aesthetic experiences do not need to be verbalized to validate their meaningfulness and significance. Regardless, I feel constant pressure to articulate artistic experiences, their felt, emotional, and sensuous qualities, and how these are embodied for purposes of learning enfolded within these involvements, for research, education, and curriculum theorizing. Ironically, as attentiveness to and curiosity towards the knowledge emerging from the arts has again gained attention from scholars, the recognition and allocation for the arts in the formal curricula at all institutional levels has further diminished. Thus, the quest to articulate sensuous, embodied, felt, and artistic knowledge in a language digestible to broader readership seems perhaps more relevant than it has in previous educational generations.

I hold a professorship in art pedagogy and my training has focused on visuals arts. However, as art forms can no longer (if this was ever the case)

Sensuous Curriculum:
Politics and the Senses in Education, pp. 175–194

be distinguished and divided by specific type, form, technique or identified to focus on specific senses, I have found myself somewhat disabled and disadvantaged in my embodied relations with others and my ability to utilize this awareness in my pedagogical thinking. When I was an art education student, we experienced a wide range of visual arts and techniques. The presence of embodied and sensuous experiences related to art was assumed but our studies did not guide us to systematically explore these aspects of knowing and being.

Much of my epistemological and pedagogical pursuits have focused on furthering my understanding of visually and artistically driven inquiries within places. I have been guided mostly by visual intrigue and perceived these place-bound inquiries as stages or scenes derived from a broader play of learning to understand. Engaged in the inquiry processes, I have mostly functioned in isolation from the physical proximity to others, people and animals, and have been rather oriented by a kind of selective relationality favoring organic materials as identifiers of and signifiers for human experiences.

Although sensuous awarenesses emerging within these places have driven the process, I have systematically suppressed the potential for sensuous relational encounters with others, people, animals, and things not immediately related to my artistic inquiry. Working with my camera within these places has been a process of affirmation of deeply felt connections as well as an entryway to exciting new understandings made possible by carefully controlled and meditative aesthetic responsiveness. However, I have recently come to understand that while this voluntary isolation from close proximity and continuous interactions with others have helped gain insights into the complex relationalities formed with organic and non-organic places and materials, adopting this orientation has also functioned as an escape from situations that have caused me discomfort in relation to people.

I believe that educators have the responsibility to continually, or at least periodically, engage in an in-depth and holistic inquiry into the motivations and values they convey and embody. I propose that the core ideas that guide sensuous curriculum theorizing as proposed by Walter Gershon in the introduction chapter of this book can be adapted to ignite and orient this pursuit. Essentially, in thinking about sensuous in the political context, Gershon articulates that understanding sensorium deeply embedded within the complex frameworks of culture and politics and "of education as sensual speaks at once to the deep histories of educational scholarship" and "is one means of enunciating this deeply layered nexus of what I call educational ways of beingknowingdoing" (p. xiii, see also Gershon, 2011).

As such, critically studying ontological, epistemological, and pedagogical beliefs and practices makes inquiry-into-knowing a holistic and sensuous practice and further necessitates rethinking how one perceives, articulates, and practices epistemology and pedagogy within the various discourses. Essentially, what I share in this chapter is part of a confessional, exploratory, and fragmented journey into the complex and varied structures of the known and non-conceptual core values that direct my professional practices, fostering or preventing sensuous curriculum from forming to reach its potential.

Against the dominant academic standard of presenting completed projects and well chewed thought patterns, I began composing this text feeling that I needed to explore and partially expose my vulnerabilities and to write from the perspective of discomfort and "insufficiency" (Blanchot, 1988, p. 8). I chose to write acknowledging my uncertainty, self-inflicted insecurity, trauma recovery, and perceived inability to fluently experience close bodily encounters. Rather than articulating my approach to sensuous curriculum from a more standard perspective of comfort and disciplined knowing established in the realm of visually dominated sensory and artistic experiences, I have exposed my impotence and dysfunctionality as an art educator. I make this text part of a "studious play" (Kalin & Barney, 2014, p. 69), a serious but playful quest towards unknown goals with only the objective of furthering my understanding of how I might be able to foster and facilitate a deeper sensuous curriculum for myself and in my interactions with others.

This text, like many others I write, presents a story of growing to understand. Partially, this is about furthering my ability to comprehend what I have already known in my feeling and sensible body but what I have not been ready to conceptualize until through this process of writing (Richardson, 1997). When I proposed this chapter, my plan was to write about the temporary connections I experience in relation to the materialized and perceived surrounding when working with and through my camera. As noted above, I have become acutely aware of my lack of sensibilities and how my relationship with my camera not only allowed me to experience unprecedented relationalities with my surrounding but also supported isolation from other people.

TOWARDS ARTISTIC AND SENSUOUS CURRICULUM THAT DISRUPTS NORMS

Thinking about the issues we face today from environmental devastation to violence, mass-migration and constant political and cultural instability, we are yet again forced to re-evaluate the value and purposes of human life. Traditionally but cyclically, the arts in education have been presented as adding an enriching aspect to human life, not as essential tools for accessing the core and foundations of all knowledge. I am amused and inspired by Kalin and Barney's (2014) critique of art education and assessment of the current practices as impotent. In my opinion, this impotence is in no small part because educators have been castrated by the endless need to adhere to prescribed, state-constructed standards, testing, and artificial regulations and expectations imposed internally and by layers of institutionalized control. Kalin and Barney use Agamben's concept of "studious play" and propose that "art educators become tinkerers playing with and transforming what is overlooked, undervalued, immeasurable, stupid, dysfunctional, and useless within the current priorities of art education, so that they may become something else" (p. 69). They further argue that "these instances of potentiality through studious play unlock our present as art educators to as-yet-undefined and uncertain futures" (p. 70).

Social justice oriented scholarship has been strongly present in the field of art education for decades. Many insightful books and collections of essays have been composed to articulate the power of arts and education to work towards more equitable and just societies, cultures, and communities (e.g., Ayers, Kumashiro, Meiners, Quinn, & Stovall, 2016; Bae & Ivashkevich, 2012; Dewhurst, 2014; Hanley, Sheppard, Noblit & Barone, 2013; Quinn, Ploof, & Hochtritt, 2011; Tavin & Ballengee Morris, 2013). Yet, over the past few decades, I have been frustrated by my inability to articulate an epistemology and define a curriculum framework grounded in a foundational sense of humane empathy, an ethical sense of relationality, and responsibility for self, others, and the planet. As a mother of two daughters, I have often pondered if it is even possible for me to raise them in a way that is less discriminatory, more fair and equitable than what I am able to conduct and conceptualize in and through my profession and everyday life.

It is well known that this kind of educational orientation cannot be achieved through non-contextual and standardized curricula founded on normative expectations for performance. Kumashiro (2000) has encouraged educators to search more broadly than educational research to look for possible ways we can build curriculum theory and practice. Arts build and foster empathetic critical understandings, and as a result, art educators in general are in position to promote building compassionate and empathetic understandings of self and others through art.

Regrettably, and contrary to this aim, the attempts have often led to more normative presentations of people and cultures in learning units. Presenting these in a manner that follows a perceived, nonoffensive neutrality and the institutional promotion of overwhelmingly normative curriculum, disables many well-intended attempts. Articulating critical multiculturalism, Acuff (2015) encourages art educators to focus less on how lessons and "things" should be conducted and to focus more on the ethical positions adopted. Bridging artistic knowing with the critical study and intentional disruption of the normative is what I believe to be significant about sensuous articulations of curriculum is this language that allows for the critical conceptualizations of holistic experiences of being in/with/through education without compromising what is fundamentally artistic, aesthetic, embodied, immediate, felt, and sensed.

My understanding is that sensory information is not raw material or preconscious data for ration and cognition. Instead thinking, feeling, believing, sensing, perceiving, and processing are simultaneous, rhizomatic, and mutually contributing processes of experiencing and understanding. These processes are not isolated and noncontextual but are instead embodied, subjective, and situational. In the introduction chapter to this book Gershon (2019) explains that

> [the ways that people make sense of the sensory information they receive are always filtered through multiple layers of sociocultural norms and values] the sensuous is inexorably political. The fields of understanding through which the sensorium is constructed and interpreted always regard questions of *whose* values are in play and what is considered normal to *whom*. Sensuous understandings therefore have material consequences. (p. xv)

It is the articulation of the sensory information and knowledge as not neutral but rather as critically and contextually framed perceptions and conceptualizations of the values that can, in my opinion, disrupt normative thinking and as a result "common sense" education (Kumashiro, 2000, 2004). Normative thinking and prevalent or disguised notions of "common sense" (Kumashiro, 2004) continue to promote and allocate marginalizing and oppressive education, pedagogy, and curriculum. Teaching for social justice towards equity and radical democracy requires interrupting normative thinking, disruption of previously unquestioned common sense. Learning that engages the sensorium (Gershon, 2019), challenges one's or a group's imagination, cognitive thinking, epistemological and ontological understandings; questions ethical motivations; gently pushes one/group to the verges of their ability to express thoughts, experiences, and emotion in written or artistic forms is perhaps the only way to truly challenge normative and pre-conceptualized thinking and reach for other possibilities.

For over a decade now, I have conducted arts-based, social justice-oriented projects at my children's schools, other schools, and in my higher education courses. I have been curious to study how children interact with one another and how, or if, they repeat their parents and caretakers' profoundly biased conscious and subconscious interactions with each other. Throughout, I have looked for openings for new understandings or subtle occurrences that would lead me to further explore the educational potential for events or encounters that may facilitate people coming together, interacting in mutually respectful ways.

IN A ROOM WITH OTHER BODIES

On weekends, I take my daughters to a community center where I attend adult dance and exercise classes daily. I have always felt a sense of belonging to this center that serves a truly diverse population, many of whom rely on service coupons and scholarships. It is not unusual for someone with whom I have never chatted with or whose name I cannot recall to inquire about the wellbeing of my two daughters or my family abroad. These incidents often occur when I feel particularly challenged by life circumstances. Community members, especially the elderly, observe and pay attention to one another, and when noticing changes in behavior, make sure that the other member feels acknowledged, recognized, and appreciated. For several years, I kept to myself and thought I was unknown to the other members—only to learn that people attending same classes keep track of one another, even when formal introductions are not made or life stories unshared.

I am not a good dancer. Yet, during these adult dance classes, I can let go and get into the beat and rhythm the way I hear and experience it. It is for this reason I have wanted my daughters to accompany me to these classes on weekends. There, my daughters too can observe and feel how bodies of different ages and abilities move to the tunes streaming from the outdated sound system blasting salsa and popular songs. They can smell, sense, and experience how people of different ages with roots and histories reaching all continents sweat and move together.

This place in particular is where I have slowly learned to reach beyond my insecurities and to be comfortable in close physical proximity with other bodies and people who are strange to me. I have never been a touchy-feely person with people outside immediate family and, living abroad far from familiar cultures and people, I have lived through periods that entailed self-imposed isolation from direct human touch and closeness. A volatile past relationship further deepened this need for physically distancing myself from other adults. Strangers, especially men, coming too close to me caused immediate experiences of anxiety. Instead, I have found safety and calm in solitude and isolation from physical closeness. Partially for this reason, my artistic practices that have framed my research and pedagogical thinking have been based on aesthetic and emotional reactions to contextual experiences dominated by vision, framed by and captured with my camera but requiring very limited physical closeness to people.

In these exercise classes I have slowly began to enjoy dancing with others. The more I have danced, the more I began to enjoy the presence of other people with whom I had no previous relationships. Beyond others' smells, the heat from their bodies, and their presence in the moments of my vulnerability (lack of dance skill), I relearned and began to relate to others in a sensuous way. Initially feeling uneasy about studying people's moving body parts and trying to mimic their movements, I slowly learned to feel their bodies-in-motion in/through mine in more holistic and sensuous ways. It gradually became more "natural" to not only mimic-and-repeat but to truly feel and sense their movements in my body, grounded in the knowledge I was gaining about mine.

My daughters have taken dance classes and in their little bodies I have observed similar rigid and task-oriented stiffness that was so familiar to me. My hope continues to be that by attending these communal exercise classes where engagement, enjoyment, and laughter dominate the dance experience that my daughters too will learn about the collective presence of people within movement, beat, and melody. And, through these experiences, eventually learn to be generous and attentive to their own bodies and, over time, to others' presence in their lives.

HUMANE, SENSUOUS PERCEPTION AND UNDERSTANDING OF SELF AND OTHERS

On a nonparticular Sunday afternoon, my younger daughter commented after class: "Mom, that one woman in the class looks exactly like you." I asked her to describe this woman as I was curious to know who she thought was so similar to me and, perhaps more selfishly, how my daughter perceived me to be. She vaguely mentioned that this woman wore similar clothes and was perhaps equally tall but she did not include many other details. So I asked her to point out the other woman next time we would see her. Weeks, perhaps even months went by and she never identified anyone. Then one day, she called me closer and said in Finnish (not to be understood by others): "Look mom, the woman who looks like you is right behind you." I looked behind me through the mirror and I smiled as this woman identified by my daughter as my look alike was much younger than I am and, if described by characteristics commonly utilized by adults, would have not been described by identifiers or attributes commonly applied to me. We had not been introduced but I had previously noted that her clothes were often similar to mine and I had always liked her presence. During class I observed her and noticed parallels in our build and our tendencies in movement.

Weeks later, a mutual friend engaged both of us in a conversation and I blurted out how my daughter thinks we look alike. I quickly added that I was flattered by my daughter's observation as she seemed much younger, was obviously very beautiful, and seemed to be athletic in ways that I was not. I could sense our mutual friend's momentary discomfort that only eased when my new friend said to me: "That's funny. I am often behind you in class and I have also noticed that we move alike and we are built somewhat alike, and I like comparing how we move."

What makes this encounter intriguing is that an adult relying on normative perceptive framework would not readily identify us two alike. This other woman is about 10–20 years younger than I am, is slightly more curvy in her build, her hair is shorter, tightly curled and almost black, and her skin is brown. My hair is blonde, my skin yellowish-pink, and my curves have years ago experienced the middle-age gravity pull towards the ground. Yet, my daughter did not think of me as belonging to a group of blonde-haired, middle aged women (no matter what their build or athletic stamina). Instead, she observed and related to my movement, my perhaps jerkier and more athletic approach to dancing, my general ways of being, and my team sports background built muscle tendencies to a woman who, by most normative classifications of identity, including age and ethnicity, does not look like me at all. My daughter did not "see" me through a peg-holed perception. She felt and sensed me amongst other dancers.

This story served as a partial opening to my daughter's thinking and was a confirmation to what I had observed in my daughters' behaviors and tendencies in describing and relating to people. More broadly, this identified some of the tendencies I have observed in my daughters' school culture among the young pupils. I regularly volunteer and often facilitate collaborative arts- and theme-based projects in their classrooms. I am there as a mother to understand my daughters' school experiences. As a researcher-mother, I am there to learn how this particular school culture makes it possible that year after year most of the students do not classify and categorize their peers, other children, and their parents according to typical census-like categories, according to sociocultural precepts such as race, gender, gender identity and expression, ableism, language, and nation of origin. Instead, the foundation of their perceptions and articulations seems to lie on a more humane foundation that is respectful of true individuality and encourages understandings of others based more on how and who they are than on sociocultural markers. This does not mean that they are unaware of concepts such as race (perceived as a historical concept) but instead that they are not categories for understanding one's peers and other people. They are not afraid of being with one another. Although how they pick their closest friends and who they associate with are kinds of personal choices based on a wide variety of factors, their language remains respectful of a person and defies normative articulations.

ARTS IN SENSUOUS SCHOOLS

Arts have the potential to complement, challenge, and question knowledge and perceptions of reality (Anttila, 2011a). Art pedagogues often work within the spirit and cultural currency of the societies in which the person is embedded and work to illuminate those tendencies. Predominantly art educators are carried by hope and working towards somewhat utopian ideals (Anttila, 2011b). This hope is born from Art's ability to foster alternative knowing and the questioning of normative thinking and education. Such an orientation to thinking ad working within the intersections of the arts and education requires constant renegotiation of curriculum and pedagogical theory and practice in order to stay true to the sensitivity to the arts and arts-based knowledge. Further, it requires a constant questioning of what the arts are as well as their role, significance, and potential in evolving cultures and societies.

Throughout my career, I have often wondered if it is even possible to raise children not to see other people and themselves in ways that are limited to and confined by the classifications of age, ethnicity, language, ableism, and so forth. As a professor of art education pedagogy, my interest has been to work with classroom teachers and children to enrich and support their curricula while also conducting practice-based research to explore the potential for context and learner focused social justice sensitive projects. Joining an arts education research group[1] that aims to create critical interventions and make broader policy suggestions has in part clarified and advanced the focus of these projects. Researchers in this group work in formal and informal educational settings with questions related to inclusion, participation, and equality. In these projects, researchers in collaboration with teachers and students design, facilitate, and study arts-based experiments and interventions. We also work together on learning projects to develop education structures and teaching practices in and through the arts and to identify institutional and cultural beliefs and mechanisms that generate and sustain unequal participation. Through this interdisciplinary research project—and in working with theater, dance, and music professionals, educators, and researchers—I have become more sensitive to the overwhelming importance of understanding how the sensorium is at the heart of our being and knowing, as well as how crucial it is to generate awareness of the ways in which everything sensuous (and everything does have its own sensuality) is also brutally political.

While facilitating collaborative projects that relate to scientific or social-responsibility themes, my interests can be articulated through the following two generative questions:

1. What kinds of artistic experiences and encounters can be utilized to further holistic and thematic learning that is deeply meaningful and might create sustainable impacts?
2. Through interactions and collaborations with various groups of children I study what fosters and supports perceptions and language that is not bound to normative categories frequently applied by adults, and what might contribute to this culture of being and learning together that resists predefinitions. Perhaps more significantly, what enables this empathetic and humane behavior in children and how can artistic and sensuous learning contribute to this within the curricula?

In sum, through experiments and analytical reflections, I aim to continuously explore (a) how sensuous and artistic approaches to curriculum and pedagogy can teach us about epistemology and (b) how might these sensuous and arts-based learning experiences further support learners already existing inclinations of ethical humanity, care, empathy, justice, and responsibility for one another, others unknowns to them, and their broader material and immaterial living contexts.

Encouraging scholars and educators to challenge and disrupt normative thinking Kumashiro's (2000, 2004) texts are an apt reminder of the dangers of normative thinking that furthers inequalities and promotes predetermined learning that sells short all education's potential to advance deeply humane cultures and flexible commons. Within the arts, there is a tradition that emphasizes apprentice-style learning of skill through repetitions and promotes learner creation stemming from educator presented "prompts."

This educational pathway presents a foundational conflict as arts are sensuous, creative, and promote imaginary learning and knowing, understandings that are dampened when forced into a form of didactic thinking that stubbornly hangs onto traditions that readily paralyze the sensuous and deeply artistic relational learning in favor of sequential linearity and singular correctness. Thus, it is relevant to return to the notions of learning that rely on norm and standard expectation, yet aim to foster the development of individual tendencies and characteristics (Saastamoinen, 2011). For example, in theatre pedagogy, Saastamoinen (2011) promotes mistakes as errors that disrupt and deviate from the norm.

To create spaces safe for mistakes and errors, much work has to enfold to build an empathetic and humane artistic learning environment that supports tranformational learning (Ellsworth, 2005; hooks,1994). In the following section, I explore some of the concepts that have helped me explore the edges of my normalized thinking, provided openings to sensuous encounters and understandings, and momentarily supported me to push myself to rethink through errors, insecurities, and insufficiency that create further openings for different kinds of articulations. My goal is to gently interrogate experiences of humane self or the learning-self (Ellsworth, 2005) in relation to bodily and artistic encounters with others. In turn, through the collaborative projects conducted in formal and informal educational settings, I aim to explore possibilities for sensuous, artistically driven inquiry in the context of ethical and political tensions, and indirectly the potential for these in advancing curriculum thinking.

PROCESS: SURRENDERING INTO BEING IN RELATION, DEVOTION, AND AVAILABILITY

As my aim is to explore the limits of my knowing I have had to rethink what research into the uncomfortable and partially unknown might entail. Thus I have returned to Laurel Richardson's (1997, 2000) *writing as a method of inquiry* and Juha Varto's (2011) *research as a non-predetermined path* to lead me to the edges of my cognitive knowing, understanding, and control. I use the term *verge* (loosely adopted from Blanchot, 1988) to articulate this search for the edges and vulnerabilities in knowing, inquiry, and self. Although not originally conceptualized in this fashion, writing this chapter was led by a self-critical exploratory process rather than a plan: it was emergent. As I worked on this chapter, I was simultaneously engaged in several school-based projects and all my writing was done in continuously evolving relations to those experiences. I have not reapplied or adopted patterns I was familiar with through my prior arts-based research processes but many similarities characterize these inquiry paths. This time, rather than writing in relation to images and my understandings emerging from them, my writing and thinking processes were guided by constant returns to moments of sensuous encounters as well as rhizomatic mashing of sensuous memories with the anticipations that emerge from this writing. By this I mean that the writing and thinking processes occurred by constantly recalling and reliving sensuous memories but also in anticipation with how the newly gained understandings will impact future encounters. I hope to articulate an attitude of *devotion,* which I believe to be the orientation that makes sensuous thinking, experiences, encounters, relations, and knowledge possible and relevant for research and curriculum theory.

Sensuous and curiously attentive presence is an attitude I have aimed to honor at every stage of this process for the potential of providing openings to immediate and reflective responsive perceptions, experiences, and notions of learning with/through/within the arts and with others. Perhaps what I am trying to share in this discussion is an orientation to language as a movement, my enthusiastic but limited communication of the ways of being that is both preliterate and simultaneously highly systematic, theorized, and analytical.

In *Becoming Animal,* Abram (2010) describes the language used by people who traditionally and primarily rely on oral communication as not definitely a "human possession, but [as] a property of the animate earth, in which we humans participate" (p. 11). There is an inherent relational and sensuous foundation in this orientation to communication. As all our thinking is based on a level of conceptualization and categorization within contexts, how do we then get to the questions that hinder on the verges or margins of knowing, those potentialities that allow access to not-yet-taken-for-granted? Everyone has their personalized and culturally learned ways and modes of operation. To get to the openings to these ethically or philosophically foundational questions I utilize the concepts of *insufficiency, relationality, devotion,* and *interface*.

Referencing Bataille, Blanchot (1988) argues the following about a principle of insufficiency/incompleteness:

> A being, insufficient as it is, does not attempt to associate itself with another being to make up a substance or integrity. The awareness of the insufficiency arises from the fact that it puts itself in question, which question needs the other or another to be enacted. (p. 5)

Led by Blanchot's writing I suggest that an awareness of insufficiency/incompleteness directs us to the other/another to evoke questions and to activate, stimulate, and contest. As Blanchot notes,

> being does not want to be recognized, it wants to be contested: in order to exist it goes towards the other, which contests and at times negates it.... The existence of every being thus summons the other or a plurality of others ... it summons a community. (p. 6)

There is a tendency to form communion, a draw toward other or another, which if committed to attentiveness and awareness leads to contention, questioning, re-questioning, rejection, and movement among people. And, perhaps, as a result, creates a foundation for *commons.* For me, utilizing various artistic and sensuous approaches has led to a series of visits or openings to the verges of my understanding and evoked this questioning and contesting of what is known or experienced in relation to the array of others. Encounters at these verges have developed a desire for a continuing, active search for such openings and are motivated by a mix of curiosity, fear, and love has in turn provoked further awareness of insufficiency of my being.

This awareness has kept me curiously alive, awakened, and somewhat alert. I cautiously understand that this awareness means a simultaneous (de)composing in relations and associations by continuously summoning others or communities of knowledge while researching for purpose continues through further collisions and reconfigurations. The path remains uncharted as with new summons and awareness comes further unreliability and unpredictability, so thus a furthered understanding of incompleteness.

All revelations or insights gained are only relevant if they pertain to life and are in some sense true to felt and lived experience (Varto, 2011, influence). I am intrigued by *radical relationality*, which, to me, means altering one's self to radical openness to various and diverse relations. While this has not meant a complete collapse of the sense of self in relation to others, places, events or concepts, it has meant willingly surrendering to processes of change one does not control or direct. This radical relationality has meant accepting that each encounter has the potential to change and/or reorganize all that I am and with who/what I am in relation with. As I assume that I am always insufficient and incomplete, despite my known self constantly changing and being altered in the flow of relations, there is no true grief, loss or sadness associated with this. While assuming radical relationality has meant accepting my inability to control relationalities, it also enables readiness and active sensuous attentiveness to seek for opening and verges for altered being.

This flexible and available sense of self has meant abandoning the notion of self as a center for thinking and agency, in as much as one can let go of one's self and nonetheless be ontologically and inevitably one's self. Applied to practice, this means exercising active openness, applauding a profound possibility and potential for change in connection to shared knowing and being—or what might be better described as the broad notion of commons—a sense of existence built upon changing commons. Scholarship is often introverted. Thoughts and developing understandings live within me for several years before being articulated. Yet, the orientation adopted here merges these polarities of individual and commons as one is simultaneously an introvert and seeking opening for merging with everything else. In writing about "devotion," Varto (2011) describes a "spontaneous thinking born out of transcendence" (p. 61) and continues: "Devotion is openness, being close to existence, spontaneity and thus the desire to let something else, the other, through" (p. 61). According to Varto, knowing and willingness or will are limited and specific, restricted ways of being in the world. Devotion, then, is rather an "intimacy with the existence" manifesting immediate and direct ties to the world. What makes this notion of being and letting be or perhaps an awareness of self as part of everything else radical, is the devotion to "non-intentionality, and non-specification" (p. 61).

Once experienced, returning to this sense of being and feeling as a sense of connectivity can become addictive. Personally, I do not perceive this a negative obsession but a form of learning to relate sensuously, artistically, and pedagogically. Through devotion or an attentive and sensuous search one is no longer indifferent but searches for access to the "interface (which) allows partial passage, because it is constantly changing" (Varto, 2011, pp. 63–64). The interface mediates multidirectional streams of information or connectivity, through which, based on my experience, bending of time and space and blending of subjectivities and perspectives becomes more readily possible. In my process of learning to understand, the encounters with others or places in the interface and their continuous recollection when writing form meaningful connections and relationalities.

Varto (2011) writes that devotion entails "being consciously intent, in surrender, in waiting" (p. 65) and continues that, "only at the interface (which includes the elements of metaxis and participation) I am in the same world with other people and the rest of being" (p. 68). Devotion as an orientation is an active alertness, readiness to return to the foundations and the beginning of knowing. For me, an orientation towards devotion means seeking opportunities to relate in unanticipated ways. I use the term *radical availability* when referring to this orientation for the reason that I am intentionally looking for change in core values and potential for renegotiating the foundations of my being and knowing. It is an attempt to expose limits and vulnerabilities and to look for verges of knowing that may provoke further interfaces with others, things, and ecologies.

RETURNING TO PEDAGOGY: SENSUOUS CURRICULUM FOUNDED IN RADICAL LOVE

I previously identified with scholarship and religious (Christian and Buddhist) writings that speak of interbeing as a mode or orientation of being that allows, and is established in, similar connectivity. *Interbeing*, entails a paradigm shift from individuality and subject based thinking, the rejection of anthropocentric views and practices and further, an adaptation of deep love, respect, and connectivity to everything surrounding us. In this context I hope that my mundane examples of being with and in connectivity with others, or struggling with these encounters, can be read as my experiences of interfaces made momentarily possible through devotion and conscious attentiveness to "sensorium" (Gershon, 2019). At the core of knowing, being present, radically available and open to change in the sense of contesting educational and political contexts and norms possible. My encounters at the interface are often brief in chronological time, a moment of connection with a child I work with for example. However, these encounters gradually 'grow' and through these encounters relationalties form and I become contested and thus face my insufficiency. Through being contested and aware of my insufficiency I then gradually form more profound relationalities that rotate the axis of my core thinking.

The story I shared from my dance class combined with the stream of brief, meaningful, and sensuous encounters initially troubled me, provoking an inquiry processes undefined by divisions of personal-professional or knowing through reason and analysis. Rather, I learned and relearned to be available and that this this availability can become a practice, a form of humane, pedagogical love. These processes require engagement with holistic learning that are not obedient to traditional Western assumptions that senses and perceptions produce pre- or raw material for cognition but that are forceful. One possible consequence of such attentions are increased holistic openings for learning that, in turn, might have the potential for more permanent changes in core values. Thus learning about and from these experiences is significant for curriculum theory.

I propose that the pedagogical significance of such artistic and incident-specific research grounded in sensuous encounters brings attentiveness to all learners' perceptions, experiences, and notions of being with one another. During the process of writing this text I have felt somewhat ill prepared to discuss the theoretical aspect of this topic as in my response to Kumashiro's (2000) call to search for alternative approaches from outside educational research I have perhaps wondered a bit far. Many argue that the separation and isolation between people and communities have diminished nature-based and environment-based natural dependencies, causing much of the violent, inhumane, and cruel behavior and attitudes that contemporary societies tolerate. This is often ironically increased through the isolation and incarceration of its most violent members as well as disproportionately and systemically pushing already marginalized peoples into jails.

Attentiveness to direct, sensuous, and corporeal daily engagements is no longer a privilege afforded to all, and perhaps never was. In addition to the works referenced before, much of my understanding about conceptualizations of presence, attentiveness, and social responsibility have evolved from Tich Nhat Hanh's books (1992, 2013, 2014), deep ecology, Vandana Shiva's (2005, 2016) writings on earth democracy and commons. Notions of radical democracy, activism, and participatory social justice, grassroots public pedagogy, as well as artistic and activist practices that aim at increased notions and policies of equity between all people, constantly reshape this foundation. Also, anarchy and anarchism have recently resurfaced as potential positions from which one is able to renegotiate societal participation and the contours of society. There are those who are willing to propose extremes in order to protect artificial borders that divide geographic locations with boundaries that split individuals and groups for inclusion or exclusion. In so doing such divisions recreate groupings of belonging and nonbelonging that are further understood to be those with guaranteed basic human rights and inherent life-value and those who do not possess these rights (Butler, 2010). I consider myself a loving human with emotional attachments and empathy not limited to those closest to me in kin or resemblance. The profoundly personal but also professional *love* I hope to articulate here entails a broad sense of connectivity and commitment to empathy. What is essential to such a love are an intent and willingness to risk one's self by being open to previously undefined relations as well as to processes and connections one cannot control or predetermine.

Stepping back a layer of scale, devotion as a pedagogical application is an empathetic and humane love grounded on sensuous knowing in the context of political tensions is an ethical act. It aims to connect and expand one's perception of what/who one is or might be by forming connections and by actively seeking participation "at one and the same basic level to everything else, to others, existence at one level in a common world" (Varto, 2011, p. 75). Its purpose is a long-lasting and ongoing sensitivity. Pedagogically, epistemologically, and ontologically this is a search for flexible foundation and the demolition of normative totality.

Devotion leads to ethical and loving relationalities through emerging interfaces and is essential because of humans naturalized tendency to discriminate and orient towards otherness through prejudice. Through the practice of devotion, one is attentive to the sensuous and returns repeatedly to the mediation that is less limited and perhaps momentarily free from this prejudice, and begins to note and adopt to the sense of much complex connectivity. For a child, like my daughter, this might be a more natural attitude. When she was learning about me, she readily utilized sensuous observations and was less limited by the kinds of normative perceptions to which other adults and I often adhere. To accomplish this, a professional may rely on studious play (Kalin & Barvey, 2014). Maybe for no other purpose but to mess around with what seems unusable, problematic or previously unnoticed. And perhaps begin through devotion begin to find new interfaces.

Sensuous curriculum to me then means to love and to love being-in-relations-with contradiction, a loving anarchy. An understanding that one' s opportunities for devotion are not readily infinite but that the impact of one's actions have infinite possibilities for participating in the formation of complex connections within the interface. Practicing and adopting the orientations of sensuous devotion and love entail care and responsibility for everything and anyone. Connectivity and humane love also entail a kind of anarchy, abandoning normative and predetermined beliefs and ways of being and opting for commons. But most importantly, this entails adopting what may be for some a radical and activist stance of resisting and/or abandoning preexisting boundaries of what and how to be, and in relations to who/what, and, eventually, a humane and caring radicalization of one's actions. Somewhat similarly, Finnish coreographer, pedagogue, and researcher Isto Turpeinen (2015) explains his pedagogical approach:

> The model is rooted in the sharing of experiences by pupil and instructor in a dialogue-based relationship. Growth and its nurturing make this possible, backed by a desire that life should be good. To lead a good life you need to build your identity and a physical and spiritual state that is yours. Concern and shared experience are important ingredients in nurturing growth in a teaching environment based on pedagogical love, or what I call an "embracing atmosphere." (p. 13)

I have been working with groups of adult and child learners for a few decades now. Learning that engages and challenges one's (or a group's) imagination, cognitive thinking, epistemological and ontological understandings, questions ethical motivations, gently pushes one/group to the verges of ability to express thoughts, experiences, and emotion in any form is perhaps the only way to truly challenge normative and preconceptualized thinking.

Awareness of one's insufficiency/incompleteness directs one toward another and evokes questions. Awareness of insufficiency/incompleteness combined with a human tendency to form communion, a draw toward other or another, when repeated can lead to the infinite contention, questioning, re-questioning, rejection, and endless movement that in turn foster holistic learning. To me, an awareness of insufficiency emerged from a series of visits or openings to or at the verge of understanding. Facilitated by a holistic sense of sensorial presence with others and within encounters evoked this questioning and somewhat radical contesting of what is known or experienced in relation to the array of others. This has led to a gradual shift towards producing knowledge as a political and value-laden activity and developing an understanding of research engagements as awareness and knowing in/as practice. Further, these processes of knowledge in the making or learning to know (repeatedly) in ways that brings forth tacit, embodied, sensorial, aesthetic, and artistic attentiveness and intentionality while also having clearly articulated emphasis on community, public or activist orientation.

Pink (2009, 2010) defines the researcher as a "sensory apprentice" when working with participants or engaging with the acknowledgement of multisensory participation. I would argue that culturally learned limitations prohibit attentiveness to sensorium and make the relearning with and working towards the potential for sensuous epistemology and curriculum difficult. But I hold on to the argument that systemic challenging of one's self in relation is not only a justified but also a foundational practice for pedagogues and scholars alike. My growth from facilitator of artful and critical learning experiences into a professional with constant, sensitive availability and attentive presence is a process (a self) in a constant making. This has been a slow process and I believe this shift takes us beyond sensory apprentice. Brief encounters with other learners in the interfaces foster radical availability and allow sensuous curriculum to emerge.

During the past few years I have learned mostly from collaborative projects and courses planned and facilitated with others. These experiences have been incredibly different in so many ways yet shared some key elements that allow transformative learning to occur. In all of these instances, a mutually identified trust and respect has been present throughout the conceptualization and facilitation in partnership. While we, my colleagues and I as well as the teachers I have worked with have planned for guiding ideas and events with great care and passion, no definite, absolute plans have been finalized and learning goals have been seen as emergent.

Throughout these collaborations, there has been constant reflection and shifts in orientation, focus, and ideology have occurred in an environment dialogue and responsiveness. What was tentatively planned has not once been completed as envisioned. I am often asked after a completion of a project what specifically was taught or what the students learned. If I were truly honest, I would state that I do not know. I rarely admit that, and I hardly ever share that we learned about being with the knowledge through the process becoming to know artfully and sensuously. Or that we learned about being together in/with the art.

An example I might share is from a classroom where I fairly regularly engage in projects with elementary students and their teachers. Ideas and frameworks for these projects emerge from the class's thematic curricula. On a surface level, one could state that we add arts-based components to complement the overall learning. While that is important, a much more meaningful relational learning has begun to emerge. As I have become more attuned with my intent and began to comprehend my role through pedagogical love and radical availability, I have been able to tune my presence to meet the children in the interface for mutual learning. Instead of working on something specific, I now orient my availability to support the learners' curiosity (theirs and mine). This might sound absurd to some but once experienced it makes perfect sense. There are often 26 students present in the room. Moving between other learning activities that occur simultaneously, students work with me based on individual interest and for the duration of their choice. Some leave after 10 minutes, some stay with me and the art for hours. I instruct them as little as possible and once they find what they want to do (for example a specific focus area on a wall size class mural) I am either quiet, listen to them talk to their peers or enter a dialogue about their work. While in the past I have struggled to surrender control, I now do it systematically with these young students. I am present and I help as needed. I touch the work with them and I attend to their process fully. I use positive encouragement and at times lead them to critical questions. People have asked what makes the projects possible as they seem daringly large and complex for students this young. Their teacher shared that she has been curious about how little direction I give and how the children so readily relate to me. Children are tinkerers engaged in studious play. Shared artistic creations provide a sensuous space to enter the interface with their learning in solo or with others. Thus it is not the students who needed to learn to know in relation. It is I who still needs to learn devotional fluency and improve my readiness for sensuous attentiveness.

NOTE

1. The author is an outside consortium collaborator in the Arts@Schools research group that is parts of the ARTSEQUAL (http://www.artsequal.fi) research initiative, coordinated by the University of the Arts Helsinki, and which examines the arts as public service, with equality as the starting point, and explores how the arts can meet the social challenges of the 2020s. The initiative is financed by the Academy of Finland's Strategic Research Council.

REFERENCES

Acuff, J. B. (2015). Failure to operationalize: Investing in Critical multicultural art education. *The Journal of Social Theory in Art Education, 35*, 30–43.

Anttila, E., & other contributing authors. (2011a). Johdanto. In E. Anttila (Ed.), *Taiteen jälki: taidepedagogiikan polkuja ja risteyksiä* (pp. 5–11). Helsinki, Finland: Teatteri korkeakoulun julkaisusarja.

Anttila, E. (2011b). Taiteen tieto ja kohtaamisen pedagogiikka. In E. Anttila (Ed.), *Taiteen jälki: taidepedagogiikan polkuja ja risteyksiä* (pp. 151–173). Helsinki, Finland: Teatteri korkeakoulun julkaisusarja.

Ayers, W., & Kumashiro, K. K., Meiners, E., Quinn, T., & Stovall, D. (2016). *Teaching towards democracy 2e: Educators as agents of change.* New York, NY: Routledge.

Abram, D. (2010). *Becoming animal: An earthly cosmology.* New York, NY: Vintage Books.

Bae, M. S., & Ivashkevich, O. (Eds.). (2012). *Girls, cultural productions, and resistance.* New York, NY: Peter Lang.

Blanchot, M. (1988). *The unavowable community* (Pierre Joris, Trans.). New York, NY: Station Hill Press.

Butler, J. (2010). *Frames of war: When is life grievable?* New York, NY: Verso.

Dewhurst, M. (2014). *Social justice art: A framework for activist art pedagogy.* Cambridge, MA: Harvard University Press.

Ellsworth, E. (2005). *Places of learning: Media, architecture, pedagogy.* London, England: Routledge.

Gershon, W. S. (2019). Introduction: Towards a sensual curriculum. Guest editor's introduction. *Journal of Curriculum Theorizing, 27*(2), 1–16.

Gershon, W. S. (Ed.). (2019). Introduction: Articulating sensuous curriculum. In *Sensuous curriculum* (pp. xiii–xx). Charlotte, NC: Information Age Publishing.

Hanley, M. S., Noblit, G. W., Sheppard, G. L., & Barone, T. (Eds.). (2013). *Culturally relevant arts education for social justice: A way out of no way.* New York, NY: Routledge.

hooks, b. (1994). *Teaching to transgress.* New York, NY: Routledge.

hooks, b. (2003). *Teaching community: A pedagogy of hope.* New York, NY: Routledge.

Kalin, M. N., & Barney, D. (2014). Inoperative art education. *Journal of Social Theory in Art Education, 34,* 64–75.

Kumashiro, K. K. (2000). Toward a theory of anti-oppressive education. *Review of Educational Research, 70*(1), 25–53.

Kumashiro, K. K. (2004). *Against common sense: Teaching and learning toward social justice.* New York, NY: Routledge.

Nhat Hanh, T. (1992). *Peace is every step: The path of mindfulness in everyday life.* New York, NY: Bantam Books.

Nhat Hanh, T. (2013). *A love letter to the earth.* Berkeley, CA: Parallex Press.

Nhat Hanh, T. (2014). *No mud, no lotus: The art of transforming suffering.* Berkeley, CA: Parallex Press.

Pink, S. (2009). *Doing sensory ethnography 2nd edition.* Los Angeles, CA: SAGE.

Pink, S. (2010). What is sensory ethnography. National Centre for Research Methods, United Kingdom. Retrieved from http://www.ncrm.ac.uk/resources/video/RMF2010/pages/18_Sensory.php

Quinn, T., Ploof, J., & Hochtritt, L. (Eds.) (2011). *Art and social justice education: Culture as commons.* New York, NY: Routledge.

Richardson, L. (1997). *Fields of play: Constructing and academic life.* New Brunswick, NJ: Rutgers University Press.

Richardson, L. (2000). Writing: A method of inquiry. In N. K. Denzin & Y. S. Lincoln (Eds.), *Handbook of qualitative research, second edition* (pp. 923–948). Thousand Oaks, CA: SAGE.

Saastamoinen, R. (2011). Prologi: Virhe taidepedagogiikan tehtävänä. In E. Anttila (Ed.), *Taiteen jälki: taidepedagogiikan polkuja ja risteyksiä* (pp. 13–16). Helsinki, Finland: Teatteri korkeakoulun julkaisusarja.

Tavin, K., & Ballengee Morris, C. (Eds.) (2013). *Stand(ing) up, for a change: Voices of arts educators.* Reston, VA: National Art Education Association.

Turpeinen, I. (2015). *Raakalautaa ja rakkautta. Kolme sommitelmaa oman elämän tanssista.* University of the Arts, Finland, Doctoral research.

Shiva, V. (2005). *Earth democracy: Justice, sustainability, and peace.* Cambridge, MA: South End Press.

Shiva, V. (2016). *Staying alive: Women, ecology, and development.* Berkeley, CA: North Atlantic Books.

Varto, J. (2011). Song of the earth. Lectures on ethics (Translated by Esa Lehtinen. Original *Laulu maasta. Luennot etiikasta,* was published in Finnish 1991/2008). Helsinki, Finland: Aalto University, School of Art and Design, Department of Art.

ABOUT THE AUTHORS

Lee Airton is an Assistant Professor of Gender and Sexuality Studies in Education at Queen's University in Kingston, Ontario. Their research program brings affect, assemblage and queer theory frameworks to bear on educational practices related to gender and sexuality in schooling and teacher education. In 2012, they founded They Is My Pronoun, a Q+A-based blog about gender-neutral pronoun usage and user support with over 30,000 unique visitors in 2017 alone. Dr. Airton also the founder of the No Big Deal Campaign, a national social media initiative that helps people show support for transgender peoples' right to have their pronouns used. In recognition of their advocacy work, Dr. Airton received a 2017 Youth Role Model of the Year Award from the Canadian Centre for Gender and Sexual Diversity. Dr. Airton's first book, *Gender—Your Guide: A Gender-Friendly Primer on What to Know, What to Say and What to Do in the New Gender Culture* offers practical steps for welcoming gender diversity in all areas of everyday life, is available from Adams Media (An Imprint of Simon & Schuster). Their scholarly publications have appeared in the journals *Gender and Education, Sex Education, Curriculum Inquiry, Teachers College Record, Journal of Education Policy* and *Teaching and Teacher Education,* and they have had editorials in *The Globe and Mail* and *The Toronto Star.*

Bernadette M. Baker is Director of Graduate Programs and a Professor of Curriculum History and Curriculum Theory in the Department of Curriculum & Instruction, University of Wisconsin, USA. Her research draws upon philosophical, historical, cosmological and sociological approaches as they inform curriculum studies, educational policy, knowledge/wisdom debates, productions of difference, processes of attachment, and enactments called culture. Her previous projects have focused on theories and analytics of power, constructions of the child, genealogies of genius, the racialization of ability and mental measurement, and the problematization of a religion-science-nation-West nexus in the making of Anglophone social sciences. Her current projects extend her interests in non-essentialist and postfoundationalist approaches, including epistemologies labeled as beyond the West, cosmologies and pedagogies informing complementary integrative health modalities, and the implications for education's present-future of discourses of vision in light of artificial intelligence, big data, educational neuroscience, and mindfulness practices. She has published widely in educational philosophy, curriculum studies, history of education, and cultural studies journals in the field.

David Lee Carlson is an associate professor in the Mary Lou Fulton Teachers College at Arizona State University. He writes in the areas of Qualitative Inquiry, Queer Theory, and Curriculum Studies. His most recent articles appear in *Journal of Curriculum and Pedagogy*, *International Journal of Research in Qualitative Inquiry*, and *Qualitative Inquiry*.

Walter S. Gershon is an associate professor in the School of Teaching, Learning & Curriculum Studies, served as Provost Associate Faculty for Diversity, Equity & Inclusion (2014–2017) and is LGBTQ Affiliate Faculty at Kent State University. His scholarship focuses on questions of social justice about how people make sense, the sociocultural contexts that inform their sense-making, and the qualitative methods used to study those processes. Although his work most often attends to how marginalized youth negotiate schools and schooling, Walter is also interested in how people of all ages negotiate educational contexts both within and outside of institutions. In addition to peer reviewed articles and book chapters, Dr. Gershon is the author of two recent award winning books—*Curriculum and Students in Classrooms: Everyday Urban Education in an Era of Standardization* (Lexington Books, 2017) and *Sound Curriculum: Sonic Studies in Educational Theory, Method, and Practic*e (Routledge, 2017).

Awad Ibrahim is an award-winning author and a Professor at the Faculty of Education, University of Ottawa, Canada. He is a Curriculum Theorist with special interest in cultural studies, applied linguistics, Hip-Hop, youth and Black popular culture, philosophy and sociology of education, social justice, diasporic and continental African identities, and ethnography. He has researched and published widely in these areas and among his books, *Provoking Curriculum Studies: Strong Poetry and the Arts of the*

Possible in Education (with Ng-A-Fook & Reis); *The Education of African Canadian Children: Critical Perspectives* (with Abdi); *Internationalizing Curriculum Studies: Histories, Environments, and Critiques* (with Hébert et al.); *In This Together: Blackness, Indigeneity, and Hip-Hop* (with Hudson & Recollet); *The rhizome of Blackness: A critical ethnography of Hip-Hop culture, language, identity and the politics of becoming*; *Critical Youth studies: A reader*; *Global linguistic flows: Hip-Hop cultures, youth identities and the politics of language* (with Alim & Pennycook).

Valerie Kinloch is the Renée and Richard Goldman Dean of the School of Education and Professor at the University of Pittsburgh. Her scholarship examines the literacies and community engagements of youth and adults inside and outside schools. Author of publications on race, place, literacy, and equity, her books include: *Still Seeking an Attitude: Critical Reflections on the Work of June Jordan* (2004), *June Jordan: Her Life and Letters* (2006), *Harlem On Our Minds: Place, Race, and the Literacies of Urban Youth* (2010), *Urban Literacies: Critical Perspectives on Language, Learning, and Community (2011), Crossing Boundaries: Teaching and Learning with Urban Youth* (2012), and *Service-Learning in Literacy Education: Possibilities for Teaching and Learning* (2015). In 2012, her book, *Harlem On Our Minds*, received the Outstanding Book of the Year Award from the American Educational Research Association (AERA). In 2014, her book titled, *Crossing Boundaries: Teaching and Learning with Urban Youth,* was a staff pick for professional development by the *Teaching Tolerance Education Magazine*. Currently, she is completing articles and book projects on literacy, equity, justice, engagement, and leadership.

Avi Lessing teaches English, coaches teachers, and directs plays outside of Chicago, at Oak Park and River Forest High School. He writes frequently about education and his essays appear in numerous journal and books. Currently he is working on a book about the need for teachers practicing relationships, in school. Avi's school is a two-time recipient of a NoVo SEL innovation grant

Carlotta Penn is an educator and daydreamer from Columbus, Ohio committed to advancing social justice in the world, especially as it relates to educational access, experiences, and outcomes. Building with diverse communities across the globe in ways that promote human rights to freedom and peace is a fulfilling and important part of her work. Her teaching and research interests are in multicultural education, literacy and language education, and critical race theory. Her research investigates how sharing personal narratives can foster opportunities for students and teachers to explore issues of identity, belonging, equity, and justice.

Kimberly Powell holds a dual appointment in the College of Education and the College of Arts and Architecture. She is an affiliate faculty member in Music Education and Asian Studies and affiliate with Arts and Design Research Incubator (ADRI) and Pennsylvania Center for Folkore. A curriculum theorist, arts educator, and educational anthropologist, her research interests include the arts as intercultural practices of identity and social inquiry, embodiment, public pedagogy, sensory and arts-based research methodologies, and. Her current research projects include *StoryWalks*, an exploration into walking methodology as an artful practice of place-making, identity, and social inquiry. She has authored or edited several publications, including *The Routledge International Handbook of Intercultural Arts Research*, and *Building Interdisciplinary and Intercultural Bridges: Where Practice Meets Research and Theory* and is co-authoring with PJ Hirayabashi a forthcoming book from Routledge about their walking research project.

Anniina Suominen is a citizen of both the United States and Finland and she has completed degrees and worked in both countries. She earned her BA/MA from the University of Arts and Design Helsinki in 1999 and her Ph.D. in Art Education from The Ohio Sate University in 2003. Since then, she has worked for Kent State and Florida State Universities and visited the University of Florida's Art Education program. She holds a position of Associate Professor of Art Pedagogy at the School of Arts, Design and Architecture at Aalto University, Finland. For the past decade and half Dr. Suominen has shared her time between the two countries navigating and negotiating their landscapes, sociocultural traditions, and institutional differences. Her simultaneous attachment to both of these geographical places has shaped her work as a scholar and an art educator. The themes she works with are conceptualized relationalities, learning in relation to place and others, gendered identities, and environmental art education, democracy and diversity art education, and visual/artistic methodologies of research.

Joseph David Sweet is an Assistant Professor of English Education at the University of North Carolina at Pembroke. His research interests include pedagogies of gender equity in secondary English Language Arts, qualitative inquiry, arts curriculum, and masculinities. Joe served as a secondary English Language Arts and theatre teacher for nine years.

Susan Uhlig is a PhD candidate in Art Education at Penn State University, where she has also served as supervisor for student teachers in art education. Prior to beginning her graduate studies at Penn State, she was a continuing lecturer in Art and Design at Purdue University where she taught numerous courses in art appreciation, art history, and art education. She continues to work for Purdue as a limited term lecturer teaching distance learning classes in art appreciation.

Boni Wozolek is currently an Assistant Professor at Penn State University, Abington College. Her work considers questions of social justice, qualitative research methods, and teaching practices that focus on the examination of race, sexual orientations, and gender identities (and their multiple forms of expression) in schools. Dr. Wozolek is the recipient of the 2012 James T. Sears Award for her paper *The Nested Nature of M/othering: Complicating Curriculum Conversations*, a 2016 Outstanding Dissertation Recognition Award from Division B (Curriculum Studies) of the American Educational Research Association, and a 2018 inductee into Kent State University's Hall of Fame for her work with marginalized populations. Recent publications include contributions to *Cultural Studies<>Critical Methodologies, The Urban Review Educational Studies,* the *Journal of LGBT Youth,* and the *Journal of Gender Studies.*

Printed and bound by CPI Group (UK) Ltd, Croydon, CR0 4YY

15/09/2026

14962335-0001